Dealing with Capacity and Other Legal Issues with Adults with Acquired Neurological Conditions

British Library Cataloguing in Publication Data

A catalogue record for this book is available from the British Library

Cover design: Jim Wilkie. Cover image: Clive Watts/Shutterstock (used under license from Shutterstock.com)

Project management, typesetting and design: J&R Publishing Services Ltd, Guildford, Surrey, UK; www.jr-publishingservices.co.uk

Printed and bound by CPI Group (UK) Ltd, Croydon, CR0 4YY

Dealing with Capacity and Other Legal Issues with Adults with Acquired Neurological Conditions

A resource for
Speech and Language Therapists

Anna Volkmer

J&R Press Ltd

It is important to note that the information contained in this book provides only an overview of the legal requirements for managing decision-making capacity and other aspects outlined in the Mental Capacity Act, 2005, within the UK. Readers should ensure they have read and understood the relevant legal framework for their location and refer to this when planning and conducting capacity assessments or any other practice related to this. They may also need to seek expert legal opinion in some cases. The authors cannot take any responsibility for readers' practice that is not consistent with the law.

Contents

Contributors

Anna Volkmer
Highly Specialist Speech and Language Therapist
South London and the Maudsley NHS Foundation Trust, London, UK

Dr Michael Dilley, MD MRCPsych
Consultant Neuropsychiatrist in Neurorehabilitation
The Wolfson Neurorehabilitation Centre
St George's University Hospitals NHS Foundation Trust, London, UK

Hannah Luff
Lead Speech and Language Therapist
South London and the Maudsley NHS Foundation Trust, London, UK

Mark Jayes
Highly Specialist Speech and Language Therapist/NIHR/HEE Clinical Doctoral
Research Fellow
Sheffield Teaching Hospitals NHS Foundation Trust/University of Sheffield

Claire Devereux
Highly Specialist Speech and Language Therapist
Sussex Partnership NHS Foundation Trust, UK

Acknowledgements

I would like to acknowledge Helena Cairney, Dr Suzanne Beeke, De Rainbow, Rhian Grounds, Jackie Bailey, Paula Volkmer and Helen Pridham for their thorough proofreading and immensely useful ideas. Also Hannah Luff, Claire Devereux, Mark Jayes and Dr Michael Dilley for their dedication and hard work to the finished product. Finally, Rachael Wilkie for her confidence and support, Kate McCabe for being my cheering squad, and James Morgan and my family for their enduring patience.

Foreword

The Mental Capacity Act, 2005, laid out for the first time a legal framework for approaching decision-making that has had a significant impact on the day-to-day care of people with neurological and neuropsychiatric conditions in the United Kingdom.

From my perspective, it is striking that, although one of the four 'tests' of capacity to make decisions is the ability to be able to communicate one's decision, the involvement of speech and language therapists in the assessment of capacity remains, on the whole, much more limited to people with aphasia, than one might expect.

Anna Volkmer, Highly Specialist Speech and Language Therapist on the Lishman Brain Injury Rehabilitation Unit at the Maudsley Hospital, has, with our multidisciplinary team colleagues, developed an approach to capacity assessment which sees the role of the speech and language therapist as central to the assessment of capacity and the subsequent management of best interests decision-making for those who lack capacity. This approach has focused our clinical service on interdisciplinary, longitudinal assessment which maximises the opportunities for different professional perspectives on how capacity may be affected, to be explored in detail and supported appropriately.

Anna's recognition of the importance of the role of the speech and language therapist in this process has led to her bringing together a number of colleagues in writing this unique book.

It brings to speech and language therapy colleagues a sharp focus on their role in capacity assessment, particularly for those with co-morbid neuropsychiatric conditions, cognitive communication impairment, impairments in social cognition and executive impairments that may have a subtle but critical impact on a person's ability to make decisions.

The day-to-day practical management of capacity assessment and best interests decision-making is often extremely complex and the provisions of the Mental Capacity Act are not always as helpful as one might hope in the clinical interventions that are subsequently made.

Here, Anna and colleagues consider novel and innovative approaches to the Act and some of the challenges which are inherent within it. They highlight how the speech and language therapist's role as not only assessor and therapist, but also advocate, enabler, educator and communicator, demands unique skills in the context of communication, which the speech and language therapist brings to the interdisciplinary approach.

It is a valuable text which acts as an excellent introduction to capacity assessment for speech and language therapists and other allied health professionals.

Dr Michael Dilley, MD MRCPsych
Consultant Neuropsychiatrist in Neurorehabilitation
Wolfson Neurorehabilitation Service
St George's University Hospitals NHS Foundation Trust, London

1 Discrimination against the vulnerable adult and their capacity to make decisions:
Do we have the skills and the time to support these people?

Anna Volkmer

Introduction

Many people with communication difficulties, and many speech and language therapists (SLTs) themselves, are passionate in stating that SLTs can be involved in the process of assessing decision-making capacity for people with communication difficulties (Mencap, 2007; ASHA, 2007; Speech Pathology Australia, 2003; RCSLT, 2014). We do this every single day when we ask our patients if we can assess them, if we can enter their homes to do a therapy session, if they would allow us to conduct a video fluoroscopy X-ray. We should not shy away from an assessment that we are more expert in than many others.

We could consider our role as championing the Mental Capacity Act (MCA, 2005) as a bill of rights for our patients. The MCA emphasises that a lack of capacity cannot be assumed. This is a bill that advocates the right of anyone who is able, including people with communication difficulties, to be involved in decision-making in every possible way, be this directly or through an advocate or attorney.

Yet SLTs are often apprehensive about assessing the decision-making capacity of their patients. This may be for a variety of reasons: perhaps because of a lack of confidence in doing the assessment, concerns about the conflict in role, or perhaps simply because there is not time in their busy schedules to prioritise this often time-consuming activity. Skinner et al. (2010) highlight that, since the publicatin of the UK Mental Capacity Act in 2005, clinicians feel worried that they do not have the experience, knowledge, training or skills to assess capacity. The authors emphasised that practicing allied health clinicians may feel that such an assessment should be the role of a specialist such as a psychologist or psychiatrist. I have met many practicing SLTs who feel this way.

This chapter considers whether there is a role for the SLT in assessing capacity, before discussing more practical issues of how this can possibly be incorporated into a routine caseload in practice, considering prioritisation and measurement of clinical impact.

Does the speech and language therapist (SLT) have a role in supporting vulnerable adults in their decision-making?

A person who lacks capacity is defined under the MCA (2005) as follows:

> "...a person lacks capacity in relation to a matter if at the material time he is unable to make a decision for himself in relation to the matter because of an impairment of, or a disturbance in the functioning of, the mind or the brain."
> (Section 2, 1)

The MCA (2005) was specifically designed for vulnerable adults including those who have had a stroke, a brain injury or who have dementia, as well as individuals with schizophrenia, delirium, concussion or suffering the consequence of drugs or alcohol use. Traditionally, SLTs provide assessment, management and intervention for adults with communication difficulties including arising from stroke, brain injury, progressive neurological conditions such as Parkinson's disease, multiple sclerosis, motor neurone disease and dementia. There are also some speech and language services in adult mental health which provide services to people with dementia and schizophrenia for example.

All of these conditions can impact on communication; on an individual's ability to understand information provided to them, remember information they have been given, to read written language, express their opinions verbally or in written form, or ask questions. In their recent response to the draft Mental Capacity Bill for Northern Ireland, The Royal College of Speech and Language Therapy (RCSLT) emphasise that speech, language and communication skills are essential for maintaining relationships, understanding social contexts, expressing individuality and exercising choice and control over personal decisions (RCSLT, 2014).

Historically, people with communication difficulties have often been excluded from decision-making, or at best had limited input. This discrimination has resulted in tragic outcomes for some of these individuals. For example, as part of their "Death by Indifference" campaign, Mencap has published in-depth case studies where this type of discrimination has resulted in the death of individuals with communication difficulties (Mencap, 2007). They suggest that much of this discrimination comes from the lack of knowledge and expertise in communication in these situations. Understanding an individual's communication difficulties and the support that may enable them to access information, as well as providing them with the opportunity and environment to get their own opinions across, requires a skilled individual such as an SLT.

The MCA 2005 Section 1 includes Principle 3, which states that "A person is not to be treated as unable to make a decision unless all practicable steps to help him to do so have been taken without success". In fact, many people with communication difficulties can demonstrate capacity to make decisions with the correct 'practical steps': communication supports. With the right communication support they are therefore able to exercise their right to choose and make their own decisions RCSLT (2014).

The MCA Code of Practice (2007) and the General Medical Council (2013) recommend seeking the professional opinion of an SLT to support capacity assessment of individuals with communication difficulties. In fact, SLTs are identified within the Adults with Incapacity Codes of Practice in Scotland (2008) as specialists in assessing and advising on capacity to understand and communicate informed decisions.

The RCSLT also advocate strongly for SLTs to be involved in assessments of decision-making capacity for people with communication difficulties. They have outlined the suggested specifics of this role in documents such as the "Submission from the Royal College of Speech and Language Therapists to the Department of Health, Social Services and Public Safety and the Department of Justice's Consultation on proposals for the Draft Mental Capacity Bill, Northern Ireland (2014)", "RCSLT Mental Health Strategy for Scotland 2011–2015: a consultation." The RCSLT has also issued a number of position papers on Speech and Language Therapy in Critical Care (2014) and Speech and Language Therapy for People with Dementia (2014) which provide specific commentary on the SLT's role in these conditions.

Table 1.1 provides a summary of these recommendations and compares them to the current known practices in speech and language therapy and the literature in these areas.

Table 1.1 Summary of RCSLT recommendations on the role of the SLT in Mental Capacity and how this fits with what is currently known about how SLTs practise in clinic and the sparse literature on these recommendations.

RCSLT recommendations on the role of the SLT in mental capacity	Case examples from the literature or current practice
"Providing an independent assessment of the individual's communication skills; their receptive and expressive language and cognitive communication difficulties, in order to provide advice on communication medium/modification requirements during the capacity assessment; identifying strategies that the individual may benefit from to understand and retain information and enable them to weigh up an issue and the aids the individual may require to make a decision and express their wishes" (Consultation on proposals for the Draft Mental Capacity Bill, Northern Ireland, RCSLT, 2014, p. 4). "SLTs have the specialist skills to assess an individual's capacity to communicate and understand information and to facilitate optimal communication. The SLT is often the person best qualified to advise on the most effective means of presenting information and choices to the person in critical care who has a significant communication disorder. This facilitates the persons' participation in their own care and decision-making process by maximising opportunity to exert free choice. This is a particularly important role for SLTs in relation to current legislation such as the Adults with Incapacity Act 2000 (Scotland), the Mental Capacity Act 2005 (England and Wales) and the Human Rights Act 1998" (RCSLT Critical Care Position paper, 2014, p. 8).	Jayes & Palmer (2013, 2014) describe how people with communication difficulties can be supported in capacity assessments using specific communication strategies. See Chapters 5 and 6 for detailed accounts of how communication can affect decision-making capacity in different conditions and a detailed description of the relevant strategies that may support people with communication difficulties.

For adults with significant communication difficulties, capacity assessments should be conducted by a 'suitably qualified person'; often the SLT may be that person (Draft Mental Capacity Bill, Northern Ireland, RCSLT, 2014).	Kindell et al. (2015) conducted a focus group of SLTs working in clinical practice with people with semantic dementia. They highlight that SLTs are conducting assessments of decision-making capacity as well as supporting people's communication skills in assessments for people with semantic dementia. Volkmer (2013) describes case examples where the SLT may be directly involved in capacity assessment, particularly when assessing an individual with dysphagia who is declining recommendations made by the SLT. See Chapters 5 and 6 for more detailed accounts and case studies.
"All staff involved in capacity assessments should receive mandatory training in communication difficulties from an SLT" (p. 6). This should include information on the mode and supports that an individual with communication difficulties may benefit from. This may include advising an appointed Independent Mental Capacity Advocate (IMCA) to enable them to communicate effectively with the person. (All from the Consultation on proposals for the Draft Mental Capacity Bill, Northern Ireland, RCSLT, 2014)	Carling-Rowland et al. (2014) demonstrate the direct impact of training social workers in communication when assessing capacity to decide on discharge destination. See Chapter 9 for a more detailed discussion on training other professionals.
SLTs may act as advocates for people with communication difficulties in the process of assessing decision-making capacity. Providing advice, training, support and the necessary aids and adaptations to those living with or caring for the person with communication difficulties such as the nominated lasting power of attorney, often the individual's family member (partner or child). These may be people who are attempting to support the person in making decisions on a day-to-day basis including choices around activities, food and therapy (Consultation on proposals for the Draft Mental Capacity Bill, Northern Ireland, RCSLT, 2014).	There is evidence that training partners who are nominated as decision-makers can maximise patient engagement. The Talking Mats© group have demonstrated the effectiveness of training carers and family members in using communication aids which can support them in understanding their loved-ones' decisions and preferences (Murphy et al., 2010). See Chapters 8 and 10 for more information on supporting communication, planning for the future and training others.

Table continued overleaf

ASHA and Speech Pathology Australia also flag the role of SLTs in advocating on the behalf of a patient and potentially serving as an expert witness in court hearings in their position papers (Aldous et al., 2014).	SLTs can have an important role in supporting testamentary capacity. Ferguson et al. (2003) provide evidence and support for this in the analysis of a case study where the testamentary capacity of a lady with aphasia is challenged following her death.
	Registered intermediaries were introduced into the UK by the Youth Justice and Criminal Evidence Act 1999; the majority of these are known to be SLTs (O'Mahoney, 2010).
	Both these examples are discussed further in Chapter 5.

The legislation around the Deprivation of Liberties Safeguards (DoLS) is currently under review and is likely to bring a new emphasis to ensuring we do not illegally detain individuals who lack capacity, an issue that has recently been raised again in the courts. These changes are likely to place a greater emphasis on assessment of capacity across all settings, and SLTs as a profession need to be prepared to deal with this.

I propose that we need to see the MCA (2005) as a document that endorses our skills as communication experts at the highest level. This document advocates our profession, and can be used in turn to advocate additional funding when developing new services or expanding existing ones. Developing a business case for new services is a complex and time-consuming process, but examples from the literature and from practice provide evidence for a more convincing business case. Case studies are provided throughout this book, but most stakeholders will be interested in relevant local evidence. Presenting cases alongside the RCSLT recommendations outlined above can emphasise the value of the care your department provides. Collecting data on current capacity assessment requests in a department can highlight a need. For example, explaining that there were 14 referrals in a 3-month time-frame and that this took x amount of time, resulting in y outcome can be useful in identifying the cost and value of this input.

Providing case examples where these services were not provided and the impact and cost implications can also be useful. Bed days and near misses can act as a warning of potential expense the trust may incur should they not provide a service. Indeed, the RCSLT position paper on critical care (2006) provides references to these costs and highlights that "difficulties ascertaining the person's capacity for informed consent and a failure to understand their preferences were seen to contribute to length of stay in intensive care settings" (p. 13). Case study 1 in Chapter 2 provides an example where an SLT was not involved and, as a result, although the individual may have retained consent capacity, treatment decisions were made without properly engaging him. This type of event is not uncommon and the "Death by Indifference" campaign by Mencap provides many more poignant examples of the real costs, besides the purely financial, that can be incurred. These types of events can result in legal cases against the organisation and can cost a significant amount of time and money. These concrete data can place a monetary value on savings that an increase in speech and language therapy services can bring.

Service level implications: Prioritising capacity assessments

In the recent past, capacity or lack of capacity was decided on the basis of a medical diagnosis alone. A person with a mental health diagnosis of schizophrenia, for example, would have been deemed to lack capacity in global terms, being viewed as unable to make any decisions. Capacity is now considered as specific to different situations (Lo, 1990). Thus there has also been a shift to a more intricate understanding of the key functional skills and abilities required for different decision-making domains.

Flew and Holly (2011) highlight that the MCA (2005) states "A person is not to be treated as unable to make a decision unless *all practicable and appropriate steps* to help him have been taken without success" (Section 1(3)). *All practicable and appropriate steps* include supporting a person's communication.

RCSLT (2014) highlighted concerns that, after the publication of the MCA Code of Practice (2007) in England, there has been an influx of referrals to speech and language therapy departments requesting capacity assessments or support in assessing people who have potential communication difficulties. This has had implications on the day-to-day management of speech and language therapy services. These are patients who may otherwise not have been referred and there are anecdotal reports of services being overwhelmed by requests. It is not only SLTs who are experiencing changes in their caseloads; psychiatrists and psychologists also report increases in time spent doing assessments of decision-making capacity (Ashby et al. 2015).

Although there may have been a sudden increase in referrals triggered by the publication of the MCA (2005) and the Code of Practice (2007) that goes with it, it is also likely that these referrals will continue to rise. Moye et al. (2004) highlight the increase in the numbers of adults surviving to older age alongside the changes in culture and finances over the last century. This has resulted in families living further away from one another and can leave older adults more vulnerable to risk. Moye et al. (2004) describe how increases in wealth in families in western societies have resulted in increased concerns around financial vulnerability and safeguarding.

Yet people with communication difficulties are being excluded from the decision-making in the process of safeguarding vulnerable adults. Communication difficulties have been identified as a significant barrier to being involved in one's own healthcare decisions (Parr et al. 1997; Knight et al., 2006). Indeed, the RCSLT 2009 Manual for Commissioning and Planning Services for SLCN, Aphasia, categorically emphasises the vulnerability of individuals with aphasia and the SLT role here:

> "Persons with aphasia remain at risk as defined by the Mental Capacity Act (2005)/Incapacity Act and speech and language therapists are integral to assessing competence for consenting etc." (p. 2)

SLTs can reduce the risks of 'negative emotional responses' such as fear, anxiety and frustration, which can fuel verbal and physical aggression from people with communication difficulties. This can be achieved by providing prompt and on-going assessment and providing appropriate communication strategies (RCSLT, 2006). In addition, if a person is able to participate in understanding and communicating decisions, they will more likely be able to, in turn, participate in their own treatment and care.

The RCSLT (2006) provides a convincing summary of the risks of not being able to engage people with communication difficulties in the decision-making process in the Adult Critical Care Position Paper:

> "Poor communication between the person who is critically ill and the physician, difficulties ascertaining the person's capacity for informed consent and a failure to understand their preferences were seen to contribute to length of stay in intensive care settings, particularly for those receiving longer-term interventions (Dowdy et al., 1998). Teno et al. (2000) reported that 'among patients who spent 14 or more days on an ICU, a substantial majority had not talked with their physicians about their preferences or prognoses'. Lilly et al. (2000) reported that 'more than 50% of patient days

were spent providing advanced supportive technology for patients that did not survive'. Increased communication with people about their values and preferences particularly related to end-of-life decisions were positively correlated with reduced length of stay (due to pro-active decisions regarding acceptance of palliative care) within the critical care environment (Dowdy et al. 1998). Hemsley et al. (2001) state that 'having a severe communication impairment could affect the length of stay for a patient as negative mood would impact on the patient's recovery or reduce the patient's ability to participate effectively in therapy".'(p. 13)

Thus, it is important that we prioritise these referrals in the same way as we would any other referral. We should be considering the risk of delayed, or no, intervention against the impact that the assessment could have. Figure 1.1 presents a prioritisation hierarchy describing how this might work in practice when prioritising SLT involvement in assessments of decision-making capacity.

The RCSLT emphasises the need to determine the prioritisation of referrals by considering both risk and the importance of timing, particularly in relation to risk reduction and health needs in Communication Quality 3 (2006). By the time this book is published, Communicating Quality Live may have been published and is likely to include further guidance in the area of capacity assessment. Balancing risks against impact is perhaps even more poignant when considering the law around decision-making capacity. The British Medical Association and The Law Society (2004) state, "Capacity is the pivotal issue in balancing the right to autonomy in decision making and the right to protection from harm" (p. 3).

Having identified the risks, how does one calculate the appropriate timing? This is likely to vary between settings and decisions, i.e. it will be dependent on the context of the decision to be made. Assessing decision-making capacity to consent to a life-saving medical procedure may be a high priority with a need for prompt action when a patient is acutely medically unwell in hospital. In comparison, an individual who is being assessed to decide on a less urgent medical intervention in the community, such as cataract surgery or a dental intervention, may not need to be seen as promptly. Similarly, an individual who is being assessed to establish his capacity to manage his finances whilst admitted to a long-term rehabilitation unit, may require less urgent intervention,

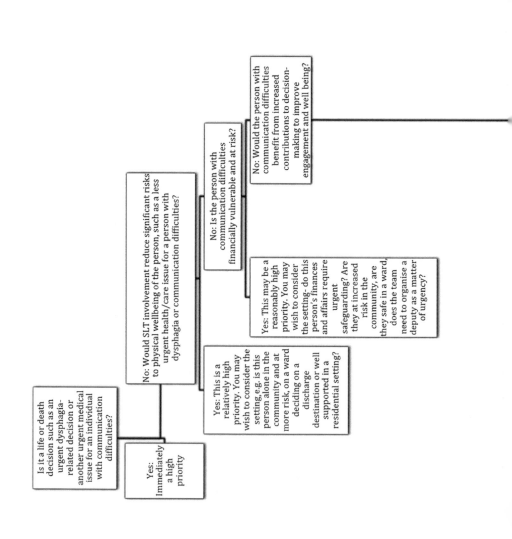

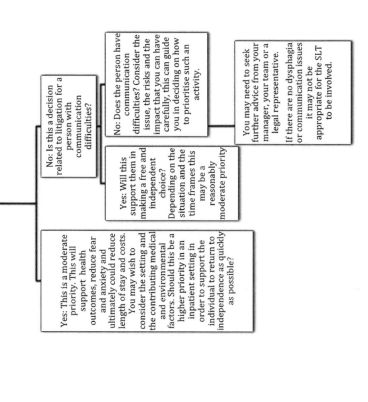

Figure 1.1 Prioritising SLT involvement in an assessment of decision-making capacity: Balancing the risks against the impact of intervention.

yet timely enough that the team can organise the consequent supports and safeguards, such as assigning a Deputy should one be required. Thus, one would argue that risk assessment requires clinical judgement to consider the individual context of the situation in question.

Some services I have worked with have considered the issues so thoroughly that they have attempted to proactively calculate risk and priorities by comparing these to the likelihood the situation would happen and the impact this could have, and in this way have identified need. This is perhaps illustrated most easily using a case study (see Case Study 1: Mrs B).

Case Study 1

Mrs B was in her mid-60s and of Caribbean descent, and had had three CVAs. Mrs B had aphasia and was known to become verbally and physically aggressive when staff or carers did not fully communicate their intentions when providing care. Mrs B also experienced visual difficulties as a result of her devastating cataracts. This caused her significant distress and often exacerbated her anxiety and aggression at night. The SLT was asked to support the assessment of her decision-making capacity to consent to a cataract operation, by attending her ophthalmology appointments with her where this was discussed. The potential risks were identified: on-going visual difficulties (high likelihood of on-going visual difficulties and thus anxiety, which would have a highly negative impact on her quality of life) and her likely reaction to staff should she not fully understand the decision or procedure (high likelihood of verbal and physical aggression, which would have a high impact on compliance, i.e. not compliant). This was compared to the potential outcomes (if supported appropriately to engage and consent it was highly likely she would happily comply, which would likely result in improved long-term vision and thus mood and behaviour). This capacity assessment was deemed a high priority for the SLT.

How can we measure the impact of our service in individual episodes of care?

> "The careful assessment of whether individuals have or
> lack capacity is essential to the protection of their rights"
> (BMA and The Law Society, 2004, p. 3).

Perhaps the best outcome of our role in assessments of decision-making capacity is the protection of an individual's rights. In health terms this may be rather a loose and difficult-to-measure type of concept. But I believe that this is perhaps the best outcome we can achieve. Can we audit the number of capacity assessments conducted with individuals with communication difficulties against the number of times an SLT was called on to support the assessment? Probably not. But perhaps we can count the increases in referral rates requesting a capacity assessment to measure success in this area. It would be interesting to know how many referrals are being made to SLTs across different services, and how these have changed. This epidemiological data could be informative to our profession as a whole, and may support service development for future generations of patients and clinicians.

Another clue to measuring outcomes is in the word 'impact'. Previous researchers have already identified length of stay, compliance, recovery and wellbeing as factors which may be improved by fully assessing and supporting an individual with communication difficulties in decision-making. It is difficult to definitively demonstrate that this type of data is linked to one intervention; there are numerous factors that may contribute to such a process. Departments can collect data on readmission, length of stay, number of risk events, discharge destination (home/residential) and diagnosis of depression in patients who have been supported to engage in decision-making. This data may be compared to patients who have ultimately been unable to engage in decision-making, thus highlighting the impact the service has had. Indeed, measures such as this are often recorded centrally and may be easy to access from internal databases. Still, proving that SLT involvement contributed to improvements is fairly difficult, particularly in a clinical setting.

The question of how to measure the impact that we have had for each individual is also challenging, and leads to topics such as satisfaction and wellbeing. Kings College Hospital (2015) uses a streaming system across their SLT service. They have identified a specific 'Capacity Stream', where they have identified any patient requiring a capacity assessment or facilitation to support a capacity assessment. They aim to deliver a specific episode of care requiring approximately 1–2 sessions of intervention. In practice, they identify outcome measurable domains in the process itself, 'the user', behaviour change and the impact. In terms of the capacity assessment process, they propose measures such as: documented communication facilitation following SLT assessment; observed or reported use of effective strategies use during the capacity assessment; provision of an informed opinion on a person's level of comprehension and expression ability in order in inform a capacity decision (in the four domains assessed in a capacity assessment). The streaming system also uses patient/carer/team satisfaction expressed in SLT strategies to facilitate process as a measure.

Both SLTs and people with aphasia themselves highlight autonomy or independence as being an important component of feeling that they are living successfully with aphasia (Brown et al., 2011). Using measures of success in participation such as goal setting or self-rating and wellbeing scores may also be useful before and after an episode of care (see Table 1.2).

Table 1.2 Summary of tools to support outcome measurement for assessments of capacity.

	Assessment tools	Descriptions
Measures of participation (i.e. participation in decision-making process)	Goal Setting: Informal goal setting or formal tools such as Goal Attainment Scaling, or the Care Aims Model	Goal Attainment Scaling (GAS) consists of a 6-step process, an interview to identify areas of difficulty and weighting of the goals from most to least important. A follow-up time is decided and the expected outcome is discussed and rated. Finally, the baseline level is documented, i.e. patient's status at time of writing goals (Bouwens et al., 2008).
		The Care Aims model is a way of "describing, measuring and representing" what a speech and language therapy service provides using eight categories of care (Malcomess, 2001). It focuses on reducing the risk and the impact of a problem. Each episode of care can be measured by reviewing the goals set in each area.

| Formal measures of wellbeing, confidence and satisfaction | Published scales such as the Aphasia Impact Questionnaire, the Visual Analogue Self-Esteem Scale or the disability questionnaire in the second section of the Comprehensive Aphasia Test

Therapy Outcome Measures (TOMs) can also be a useful therapist-rated measure of outcomes | The Aphasia Impact Questionnaire (Swinburn et al., 2012) asks questions about living with aphasia and how people feel, how confident they are and how they feel they are coping. Individuals are asked to rate these areas before and after they have engaged in an intervention.

The Visual Analogue Self-Esteem Scale (Brumfitt & Sheeran, 2010) is a measure of self-esteem designed to be used with people with aphasia and communication difficulties. It asks individuals to rate how they feel about their communication and can be used as an outcome measure.

The Comprehensive Aphasia Test (CAT) (Swinburn et al., 2004) includes a disability questionnaire that explores the practical, psychological and social impact of aphasia and communication difficulties from the perspective of the person with aphasia themselves.

Therapy Outcome Measure (TOMs Updated, Enderby & John, 2015) allows the SLT to rate the areas of impairment, activity, participation and wellbeing on an 11-point ordinal scale in order to measure changes over time. |
| Informal measures of satisfaction and wellbeing | PROMS/FROMS or informal, therapy designed rating methods | Patient Reported Outcome Measures (PROMS) or Family Reported Outcome Measures (FROMS) are increasingly being used in the NHS. Collecting relevant data as part of an episode of care, for example, ticking boxes in response to questions, or rating themselves on a scale on either paper-based or computerised systems can yield pertinent and valuable data to enhance a service (Nelson et al., 2015). These are perhaps the most achievable measures that can be collected as part of the capacity assessment process. |

Summary

Managing referrals for capacity assessments is a relatively novel area for us as SLTs. But it is now becoming a routine part of our role in day-to-day clinical practice. The four cornerstones of capacity assessments –understanding, retaining, weighing up and communicating – are in some ways our bread and butter as SLTs. These are areas in which we are already skilled in assessing and evaluating our patients.

What is perhaps more challenging within our services is finding the resources amongst our other responsibilities. Supporting and conducting capacity assessments will need to be prioritised and measured. Patients could be prioritised by considering the risks and timeliness, as recommended by the RCSLT (2006). And perhaps some of these risks can in turn be measured through audit to provide data on the impact the service is having. On a more individual basis, gathering feedback from patients using measures such as goal setting or satisfaction measures will also yield valuable information. In the current political climate of National Health Service (NHS) austerity, we urgently need more information in this area of clinical practice.

The Mental Capacity Act (2005) could be seen as a 'Bill of Rights' for people with communication difficulties. It is a vehicle to protect the independence of our patients and justify expansion of speech and language therapy services to provide this support across expanding caseloads of people with dementia, stroke, brain injury, and progressive neurological conditions as well as any other vulnerable adults with communication difficulties.

References

Aldous, K., Tolmie, R., Worrall, L. & Ferguson, A. (2014) Speech-Language Pathologists' contributions to the assessment of decision-making capacity in aphasia: A survey of common practices. *International Journal of Speech-Language Pathology*, 16(3): 231–241.

ASHA (2007) *Scope of Practice in Speech-Language Pathology*. Rockville Pike, MD: American Speech-Language-Hearing Association.

Ashby, G.A., Griffin, C. & Agrawal, N. (2015) Brain injury and deprivation of liberty on neurosciences wards: 'A gilded cage is still a cage'. *Practical Neurology*, 15(5): 361–368.

Bouwens, S.F.M., van Heugten, C.M. & Verhey, F.R.J. (2008) Review of goal attainment scaling as a useful outcome measure in psychogeriatric patients with cognitive disorders. *Dementia and Geriatric Cognitive Disorders*, 26, 528–540.

British Medical Association and The Law Society (2004) *Mental Capacity: Guidance for Doctors and Lawyers*, 2nd ed. London, BMJ Books.

Brown, K., Worrall, L., Davidson, B. & Howe, T. (2011) Exploring speech–language pathologists' perspectives about living successfully with aphasia. *International Journal of Language and Communication Disorders*, 46(3): 300–311.

Brumfitt, S. & Sheeran, P. (2010) *Visual Analogue Self-Esteem Scale*. UK, Speechmark Publishing Ltd.

Carling-Rowland, A., Black, S., McDonald, L. & Kagan, A. (2014) Increasing access to fair capacity evaluation for discharge decision-making for people with aphasia: A randomized controlled trial. *Aphasiology*, 28(6): 750–765.

Enderby, P. & John, A. (2015) *Therapy Outcome Measures for Rehabilitation Professionals*, 3rd ed. Guildford, J&R Press.

Ferguson, A., Worrall, L., McPhee, J., Buskell, R., Armstrong, E. & Togher, L. (2003) Case Study: Testamentary capacity and aphasia: A descriptive case report with implications for clinical practice. *Aphasiology*, 17(10): 965–980.

Flew, R. & Holly, C. (2011) Has the Mental Capacity Act changed the way SLTs work? Conference Presentation at RCSLT Wales Board Professional Development Day: Best Practice in Delegation.

General Medical Council (2013) Good Medical Practice. http://www.gmc-uk.org/guidance/ethical_guidance/consent_guidance_accessing_capacity.asp

Jayes, M. & Palmer, R. (2013) Initial evaluation of the Consent Support Tool: A structured procedure to facilitate the inclusion and engagement of people with aphasia in the informed consent process. *International Journal of Speech-Language Pathology*, 1–10. DOI: 10.3109/17549507.2013.7959999

Jayes, M. & Palmer, R. (2014) Stroke research staff's experiences of seeking consent from people with communication difficulties: Results of a national online survey. *Topics in Stroke Rehab*, 21(5): 443–451.

Kindell, J., Sage, K., & Cruice, M. (2015) Supporting communication in semantic dementia: Clinical consensus from expert practitioners. *Quality in Aging and Older Adults*, *16*(3), 153–164.

Kings College Hospital Speech and Language Therapy Department (unpublished, 2015) Care Streams.

Knight, K., Worrall, L. & Rose, T. (2006) The provision of health information to stroke patients within an acute hospital setting: What actually happens and how do patients feel about it? *Top Stroke Rehabilitation*, 13(1): 78–97.

Lo, B. (1990) Assessing decision-making capacity. *Law, Medicine and Health Care*, 18: 193–201.

Malcomess, K. (2001) The reason for care. RCSLT *Bulletin* 595, November: 12.

Mencap (2007) Death by Indifference (viewed June 2015) https://www.mencap.org.uk/sites/default/files/documents/2008-03/DBIreport.pdf

Mental Capacity Act 2005: http://www.legislation.gov.uk/ukpga/2005/9/pdfs/ukpga_20050009_en.pdfThe Mental Health Act 2005

Mental Capacity Act 2005 Code of Practice (2007): http://www.legislation.gov.uk/ukpga/2005/9/pdfs/ukpgacop_20050009_en.pdf

Moye, J., Karel, M.J.M., Azar, A.R. & Guerrera, R.J. (2004) Capacity to consent to treatment: Empirical comparison of three instruments in older adults with and without dementia. *The Gerentologist*, 44(2): 166–175.

Murphy, J., Oliver, T.M. & Cox, S. (2010) Talking Mats and involvement in decision making for people with dementia and family carers: Full Report. Joseph Rowntree Foundation. www.jrf.org.uk Downloaded from: http://www.jrf.org.uk/sites/files/jrf/Talking-Mats-and-decision-making-full.pdf

Nelson, E., Eftimovska, E., Lind, C., Hager, A., Wasson, J.H. & Linbald, S. (2015) Patient reported outcome measures in practice. *BMJ*, 350: g7818.

O'Mahoney, B. (2010) The emerging role of the Registered Intermediary with the vulnerable witness and offender: Facilitating communication with the police and members of the judiciary. *British Journal of Learning Disabilities*, 38(3): 232–237.

Parr, S., Byng, S. & Gilpin, S. (1997) *Talking about Aphasia*. Buckingham, Open University Press.

Royal College of Speech and Language Therapy (RCSLT) (2006) Communicating Quality 3. Scotprint. UK.

Royal College of Speech and Language Therapy (RCSLT) (2006) Position Paper: Speech and Language Therapy in Adult Critical Care. London, RSCLT.

Royal College of Speech and Language Therapy (RCSLT) (2009) Manual for Commissioning and Planning Services for SLCN, Aphasia. http://www.rcslt.org/members/docs/aphasia_resource_updatedfeb2014

Royal College of Speech and Language Therapy (RCSLT) (2014) Position Paper: Speech and Language Therapy in Adult Critical Care. http://www.rcslt.org/members/publications/publications2/criticalcare_positionpaper_060114

Royal College of Speech and Language Therapy (RCSLT) (2014) SLT Provision for People with Dementia: RCSLT Position Paper. http://www.rcslt.org/members/publications/publications2/dementia_position_paper2014

Royal College of Speech and Language Therapy (RCSLT) (2014) Submission from the Royal College of Speech and Language Therapists to the Department of Health, Social Services and Public Safety and the Department of Justice's Consultation on proposals for the Draft Mental Capacity Bill, Northern Ireland. http://www.rcslt.org/governments/docs/draft_mentalcapacity_bill

Royal College of Speech and Language Therapy (RCSLT) Mental Health Strategy for Scotland 2011–2015: A consultation. http://www.scotland.gov.uk/Resource/0045/00450338.pdf

Scottish Government (2008) Revised Code of Practice. For persons authorised under intervention orders and guardians. Scotland. RR Donnelley. http://www.gov.scot/Resource/Doc/216558/0058064.pdf

Skinner, R., Joiner, C., Chesters, L., Bates, L. & Scrivener, L. (2010) Demystifying the process? A multidisciplinary approach to assessing capacity for adults with a learning disability. *British Journal of Learning Disabilities*, 39, 92–97.

Speech Pathology Australia (2003) *Scope of Practice in Speech Pathology*. Melbourne, Australia.

Swinburn, K., McVicker, S. & Cruice, M. (2012) Measuring outcomes in community services: Patient reported outcome measurement for people with aphasia. *International Journal of Stroke*, 7(suppl2), 30. DOI: 10.1111/j.1747-4930.2012.00961.x

Swinburn, K., Porter, G. & Howard, D. (2004) *Comprehensive Aphasia Test (CAT)*. Hove: Psychology Press.

Volkmer, A. (2013) *Assessment and Therapy for Language and Cognitive Communication Difficulties in Dementia and Other Progressive Diseases*. Guildford: J&R Press.

2 Demystifying the Mental Health Act and Mental Capacity Act: What is capacity?

Anna Volkmer

> "Mental capacity means a person's ability to make their own choices and decisions. Under UK law, someone's capacity is judged according to the specific decision to be made, so a person may have sufficient capacity to make simple decisions but not more complicated ones" (Sense Website, viewed September 2015).

Introduction

The Mental Capacity Act (MCA) 2005 was given Royal Assent in April 2005 and came into force in 2007. It covers individuals aged 16 or over in England and Wales. It does not cover Scotland or Northern Ireland. Scotland has The Adults with Incapacity Act 2000 which sets out in law a range of options to help people aged 16 or over who lack the capacity. Scotland also has an Office for the Public Guardian. Northern Ireland does not currently have a capacity act but is currently examining and writing its laws for people who lack capacity (in the forthcoming Mental Capacity Bill).

The MCA (2005) has set out the current laws to protect and empower people who may lack capacity in England and Wales. It is a landmark document which health professionals should be familiar with. The MCA (2005) can be accessed for free online (see Useful Resources at the end of this book) and is accompanied by a Code of Practice, published in 2007. The Code of Practice (2007) provides guidance and information about how the MCA (2005) works in practice on a day-to-day basis, and includes examples of how this might happen.

This chapter summarises some of the history surrounding mental health and the complementary law to protect vulnerable adults that preceded and influenced the current mental capacity legislation. This will provide the necessary context to better understand the thinking behind the MCA (2005). We will discuss the discrimination that many of our patients would have faced in the past and how the current MCA (2005) aims to reduce the risk of this occurring again. This chapter then goes on to describe the areas of the current MCA (2005) that are most relevant to us as speech and language therapists (SLTs). These are illustrated with case studies that have been contributed from SLTs across different service settings.

Lunatics and madhouses: Mental health in Britain over the last 300 years

Much of the law protecting vulnerable adults was shaped or influenced by the laws that protect adults with mental health conditions. Indeed, in the not too distant past and still today there is a significant lack of understanding about mental and many physical health conditions that impact on thinking, cognition and behaviour. Most SLTs can recall examples of discrimination toward their patients, for example, people with dysarthria being presumed to be drunk, and people judging aphasics who are unable to communicate verbally as stupid or deaf and not asking them questions, instead deferring to others around them or making choices on their behalf.

Thus people have been discriminated against and judged without consideration of their actual abilities or their rights as human beings. These rights include the right to freedom, to health care and perhaps, most importantly for this discussion, the right to choose, if able. As society and medicine has come to better understand mental and physical health so has the law protecting these people changed. The following provides a brief summary of the development and major changes in Mental Health legislation over the last 300 years or so.

1700's Many of us may have read Charlotte Bronte's novel Jane Eyre, set most likely in the late 1700s or early 1800s. The novel describes how one of the central figures, Mr Rochester, locks his wife up in the attic as she descended into 'madness'. Indeed, by the middle of the 17th century the most common way to deal with mentally unwell family members was to keep them at home, often out of sight, or to pay to have them kept in a type of private boarding house or 'madhouse'. No medical diagnosis was required; in fact, it seems that not even lists were kept nor standards maintained or monitored in these types of institutions. Thus people could be locked up who were quite well. Some accounts suggest that many sane people (often women) were locked up by relatives who kept up payments; imprisoning them against their will. In addition, the conditions in these institutions were described as 'atrocious'.

1774 In 1763, a Select Committee of the House of Commons was set up to study the problem. This led to **The Madhouses Act 1774** and provided physicians with powers to grant licenses to premises housing 'lunatics' in London. People were only admitted to these 'madhouses' with a certification signed by a doctor.

1845 In 1845, **The Lunacy Act** and the **County Asylums Act** together gave mental hospitals or 'asylums' the authority to detain "lunatics, idiots and persons of unsound mind". This meant that people with mental illness were now considered 'patients' who required treatment and care.

1890 Both these acts were replaced by the **Lunacy Act 1890**. This act introduced 'reception orders' which were required in order to detain someone in an asylum. These orders were specific, requiring an assessment by two medical professionals and the raising of a petition to a judicial authority before a person could be admitted. The order would be made by a specialised Justice of the Peace and lasted one year. After this period, detention could be renewed at regular intervals by submission of a medical report to the Lunacy Commission.

1913 The **Mental Deficiency Act 1913** renamed the Lunacy Commission as the 'Board of Control' and increased the range of its powers. The functions of the Board of Control were further changed by
1930 the **Mental Treatment Act 1930**.

1959 Following the introduction of the National Health Service Act in 1946 a new **Mental Health Act 1959** replaced those that had gone before. Consistent with the medical focus of the Macmillan Commission which endorsed the idea that both mental and physical health are medical conditions, this act aimed for the provision of informal treatment for the majority of people suffering from mental disorders. This legal framework outlined that people were only detained in hospital if absolutely necessary. The act also abolished the involvement of the magistrate in detaining individuals, handing this power to the health professionals.

1983   Twenty-four years later the Mental Health Act was revised and **The Mental Health Act 1983** came into effect in September that year. It included legislation for the use of treatments such as psychiatric medications, electroconvulsive therapy and psychosurgery. Specifically, it provided the legislation that allowed people diagnosed with a mental disorder to be detained in hospital or police custody and have their disorder assessed or treated against their wishes. This is now unofficially known as 'sectioning'. The Mental Health Act 1983 applied to people in England and Wales and provided guidance on the admission, care and treatment of mentally disordered persons, as well as other complex issues such as the management of their property.

1997   A new Mental Health Bill was again under discussion between 1997 and 2006. At this time, many psychiatrists and social commentators publicly expressed concerns that the changes proposed by a new Mental Health Bill were draconian. Many criticised the changes and attributed these modifications to increasing government and media concern about the consequences of deinstitutionalisation:

> "The perception was that the closing of the old asylums meant that people with mental illnesses were inadequately contained and were putting the community at risk." ... "Having professionalised the process of dealing with the mad in 1959, the Government now appears to be clawing back power to itself, in the belief that psychiatrists are not locking enough people up" (Moncreiff, 2003, p. 8–9).

In the meantime, the Mental Capacity Act (MCA) was given Royal Assent in April 2005, before it came into force later in 2007 (the development of this act is described later in this chapter). The MCA (2005) complemented the Mental Health Act.

2007/   In 2006 the government was forced to abandon its original plans
2008   to introduce a new Mental Health Bill outright and instead amended
              the 1983 Act. Despite this, the Bill was still defeated a number of
              times in the House of Lords prior to its receiving Royal Assent.
              The Mental Health Act 2007 amends the Mental Health Act 1983.
              Most of the Act was implemented in November 2008. The changes
              notably included the introduction of the Mental Health Review
              Tribunal, or hearings, which aim to improve patient safeguards by
              allowing individuals to challenge their admissions. The tribunals
              are empowered by law to adjudicate disputes about mental health
              treatment, mainly by conducting independent reviews of patients
              detained in psychiatric hospitals, or under outpatient commitment,
              and who may be subject to involuntary treatment.

(Compiled with information collected from: National Archives Website; an article on The Mental Health Foundation website written by Lawton-Smith and McCulloch [Mentalhealthcare.org.uk website]; Mental Health Act 1983: An outline guide. A useful summary of the Act from 'Mind' (all viewed 2015); Mental Health Act 1959; Mental Health Act 2007; Moncreiff (2003)).

Past to present: Protecting vulnerable adults in England and Wales

In the past, the laws protecting vulnerable adults often focused more on the financial aspects of their day-to-day lives. As medicine has advanced, society has become older and richer and families don't always live so close to one another. This has meant that financial capacity has become an even greater concern to our patients and their family members. We have also developed a better understanding of other types of decision-making such as consent to treatment, placement issues and testamentary capacity. This area of health research will likely continue to develop and broaden our understanding of the cognitive skills involved in decision-making.

The law has also had to change to accommodate these developments. Legal decision-making practices in this area are based on both common law and statutory law. Common law describes the part of English law which is not based on an Act, but on previous cases: judicial precedent. Statutory law is based on written primary legislations and statutory instruments such as the Mental Health Act itself. Often, common law (case decisions) will influence the interpretation, development or modifications of new Acts. This is important for us as clinicians. It may be that an issue we are concerned about has not been 'covered' by the MCA (2005). In these cases, consulting with the specialist teams within the organisation, including the legal team, can be useful, as well as looking at what has previously happened in the relevant law. Many of the more high-profile cases can reach the media, particularly those related to end-of-life and, occasionally, feeding issues. The Internet can also provide a resource for accessing the media surrounding these types of cases (see Useful Websites listed under Useful Resources at the end of this book).

The following provides a summary of the history surrounding mental capacity and the laws protecting individuals who lack capacity:

Pre-1959 In the past, the issue of making decisions was only of concern if the incapacitated individual owned a certain amount of property. Up until 1959, the principles of '*parens patriae*' provided the legal basis for surrogate decision-making on behalf of '*non compos mentis*' adults. The first expression (which literally means 'the parent of the country') refers to the Crown's power and duty to protect the persons and property of those unable to do so for themselves, including minors and adults of unsound mind.

If the person was considered not of sound mind for the purposes of administering or disposing of their property, the Crown would take charge of their property and possessions as well as deciding on their care. The property of 'idiots' and 'lunatics' was the responsibility of the Lord Chancellor. These people were sometimes known as 'Chancery lunatics'. The Crown was entitled to administer the lands of an 'idiot' during his life, but of the 'lunatic' only during periods of insanity. The lands or possessions were normally granted out for the duration of the 'lunacy' or 'idiocy' to 'committees' (in other words, those to whose care the 'lunatic' or their estate was committed).

In general, people who brought 'lunatics' and 'idiots' to the Chancellor's attention had a particular interest, such as relatives, solicitors, or others acting as the executors of a will. In order to make such a request, at least two sworn affidavits had to be submitted supporting their opinion of the state of mind of the supposed 'lunatic'. 'Lunatics' were considered globally to lack capacity to manage their affairs.

1959   After 1959, the *'parens patriae'* jurisdiction gave way to the regulations of the Mental Health Act. This Act instructed that "the judge may, with respect to the property and affairs of a patient, do or secure the doing of all such things as appear necessary or expedient [...] for making provision for other persons or purposes for whom or which the patient might be expected to provide it were he not mentally disordered" (section 102 (1) (c)). This statement formed the statutory basis for the substituted judgement test. The idea of the substituted judgement test had already been evident in earlier cases, for example in 1816 in the case of *Re Hinde, ex parte Whitbread*. In this case, Lord Eldon proposed that "the Court, looking at what it is likely the Lunatic himself would do, if he were in a capacity to act, will make some provision out of the estate for those persons". The Court provided an allowance to the man's siblings "upon the principle that it would naturally be more agreeable to the lunatic, [...] than that they should be sent into the world to disgrace him as beggars".

The substituted judgement test was further refined after 1959 in common law. There was a case at this time, *Re L (WJG)*, which introduced the idea that a patient could have a hypothetical 'brief lucid interval'. The person's decision-making in these 'intervals' should guide the process of substituted decision-making. For this, the judge had to "assume that the patient becomes a sane man for a sufficient time to review the situation but knows that after a brief interval of sanity he will once more be as he was before". More recently, commentators and researchers emphasised that the substituted judgement standard may also be overused in some cases (Szerletics, 2012). Szerletics (2012) highlighted the case of Re C where the court advised that if the person has never had capacity before, then the Court shall assume that the patient would have been "a normal decent person, acting in accordance with contemporary standards of morality".

Notably, the Mental Health Act of 1959 did not provide any advice on the management of non-financial affairs, such as welfare and medical procedures. The previous legislation based on the principles of *'parens patriae'* had enabled the court to make decisions related to these issues. Thus a gap was created. It was not until 1990 that real actions were taken to consider issues of capacity outside of financial affairs. This was when the concept of 'common law necessity' was considered in case law. This changed as a result of a case brought 1990 where the House of Lords used this principle to defend the actions taken in the sterilisation of a handicapped woman. From this point, in case law, a medical intervention or act could be considered lawful if it were deemed necessary for life and limb. For example, if to save someone's life following an accident, a person needed to undergo surgery even though they were unconscious and the medical practitioner couldn't gain consent, then this would be considered lawful. Unfortunately, this principle did not cover all welfare-related decisions, such as where the best place to live for an individual might be. Indeed, family judges ended up reinventing the ideas of '*parens patriae*' in court to support decisions such as protecting vulnerable children from returning to abusive families. One example of this was in a landmark case in 2000, Re F, where the courts prevented a child returning to live with her abusive natural mother.

1990   In 1990, the principles of 'common law necessity' described above were complemented by the introduction of the Bolam test. This was adopted by the High Court and often used in defence of alleged medical negligence as well as in supporting best interests decisions. The Bolam test proposed that if there is a body of evidence or expertise to support the decision made by that practitioner then it is a lawful decision, even if there is another group who would not have done so. So for example, when considering whether to continue or withdraw artificial nutrition from a patient in a persistent vegetative state, there is a considerable body of opinion supporting the notion that it is not in the person's best interests to be kept alive no matter the cost, as in the case of *Airedale NHS Trust v Bland*.

The Bolam test has since been called into question as it only really considers the medical best interests of an individual, not the emotional, social or other welfare needs of the individual. In fact, the paternalistic notion that the doctor knows best was challenged in the case of *Re SL* regarding the sterilisation of a 29-year-old mentally incapacitated woman. The judge in this case highlighted that both sterilisation by total hysterectomy and use of a contraceptive coil were equally lawful due to the split of medical opinion on the use of either of these techniques as effective. Yet, considering that the latter was the least invasive, this could perhaps be considered 'in the best interests' in terms of the broader best interests of the individual. In short, the Bolam test, although a valuable point, is no longer a complete test of best interests.

Since then, the concept of best interests has been developed to incorporate many more principles. These include both physical welfare (health, care needs and consistency) as well as emotional needs, importance of relationships and sense of belonging. These principles can balance what might be safest with what might make someone happiest. Yet the substituted judgement standard and best interest decisions can be considered separate and complementary concepts. What is in a 'person's best interests' may not need to be considered if there is an idea of what that person decided when lucid.

2005   The Mental Capacity Act (MCA) came into statutory law in 2005. The MCA considered the issues of the substituted judgement standard and best interests decisions in great detail. The MCA provides a detailed checklist on how to assess capacity to make a decision and whether an individual requires a best interests decision to be made for them. The MCA guides current legal and health-related decision-making and applies to both financial decision-making as well as welfare, medical consent and other issues. The following provides a more detailed description of the MCA.

(Compiled with information collected from: The National Archives Website; an article on The Mental Health Foundation Website by Lawton-Smith & McCulloch [Mentalhealthcare.org.uk]; Mental Health Act 1983: An outline guide. A useful summary of the Act from 'Mind', (all viewed 2015); Mental Health Act 1959; Mental Health Act 2007; Szerletics (2012); as well as information from the following cases including *Re Hinde, ex parte Whitbread (1816)*, *Re Airedale NHS Trust v Bland* (1861); *Re SL* (2000); *Re F* (2001) and *Re L (WJG) (1966)*.)

The Mental Capacity Act 2005:

The Mental Capacity Act (MCA, 2005) is divided into three major sections:

Part 1 Persons who lack capacity

Part 2 The Court of Protection and the Public Guardian

Part 3 Miscellaneous and General

Each of these section deals with various aspects of capacity. Part 1 emphasises the principles of the MCA (2005) and then outlines descriptions of 'Persons who lack capacity' and 'Inability to make decisions'. Parts 2 and 3 also describe new roles, bodies and powers (Lasting Power of Attorney, LPA), Court of Protection and Independent Mental Capacity Advocates (IMCA). For the purposes of assessing decision-making capacity, Part 1 is perhaps the most significant section of the MCA. However, it is valuable to understand the remaining sections, such as LPA, in order to advise and support patients and their relatives who may need advice and training in how best to communicate with their loved ones in order to support the decision-making process. Similarly, IMCAs may be called upon to represent our patients' views and may benefit from training and advice from an SLT.

Some of the main points from Part 1 of the MCA (2005) are outlined in Table 2.1.

Table 2.1 Fundamental concepts from Part 1 of the MCA (2005).

Fundamental concepts to support the assessment of decision-making capacity from the Mental Capacity Act 2005
Principles
A person must be assumed to have capacity unless it is established that he lacks capacity.
A person is not to be treated as unable to make a decision unless all practicable steps to help him to do so have been taken without success.
A person is not to be treated as unable to make a decision merely because he makes an unwise decision.
An act done, or decision made, under this Act for or on behalf of a person who lacks capacity must be done, or made, in his best interests.
Before the act is done, or the decision is made, regard must be had to whether the purpose for which it is needed can be as effectively achieved in a way that is less restrictive of the person's rights and freedom of action.

Persons who lack capacity

For the purposes of this Act, a person lacks capacity in relation to a matter if at the material time he is unable to make a decision for himself in relation to the matter because of an impairment of, or a disturbance in the functioning of, the mind or brain.

It does not matter whether the impairment or disturbance is permanent or temporary.

A lack of capacity cannot be established merely by reference to–

(a) a person's age or appearance, or

(b) a condition of his, or an aspect of his behaviour, which might lead others to make unjustified assumptions about his capacity.

In proceedings under this Act or any other enactment, any question whether a person lacks capacity within the meaning of this Act must be decided on the balance of probabilities.

Inability to make decisions

For the purposes of section 2, a person is unable to make a decision for himself if he is unable–

(a) to understand the information relevant to the decision,

(b) to retain that information,

(c) to use or weigh that information as part of the process of making the decision, or

(d) to communicate his decision (whether by talking, using sign language or any other means).

A person is not to be regarded as unable to understand the information relevant to a decision if he is able to understand an explanation of it given to him in a way that is appropriate to his circumstances (using simple language, visual aids or any other means).

The fact that a person is able to retain the information relevant to a decision for a short period only does not prevent him from being regarded as able to make the decision.

The information relevant to a decision includes information about the reasonably foreseeable consequences of–

(a) deciding one way or another, or

(b) failing to make the decision.

Principles of the Mental Capacity Act (2005)

Capacity is defined as the ability to do something. In legal terms, this includes the person's ability to make a decision which may have legal consequences for that person or for others (British Medical Association and The Law Society, 2004). The BMA and The Law Society (2004) state that: "The law is clear; all adults are presumed to have legal capacity unless there is evidence to the contrary" (p. 5). This sentiment forms the first of the principles of the MCA (2005). In the case of people with communication difficulties such as aphasia or dysarthria, there may be immediate evidence that suggests an individual may not have capacity to make a decision. A person with a communication difficulty may be more likely to be expected to prove their capacity than someone without communication difficulties. A nurse specialist recently highlighted to me that if an individual such as Stephen Hawking were admitted to hospital it would be unlikely that staff would judge his nonverbal communication as a signal that he lacks the capacity to make decisions, for he has demonstrated his capacity by being Stephen Hawking. Not many have this luxury.

It is not uncommon for staff to question an individual's capacity for decision-making due to their evident communication difficulties. Importantly, in this situation it should not be assumed that the individual lacks capacity; an assessment should be conducted at this point, using appropriate aids to support communication. This is where the team will benefit from the advice of an SLT. An SLT is the expert clinician in the areas of receptive and expressive language, which comprise two points of the capacity assessment; namely, understanding information and communicating a decision. The MCA (2005) emphasises that an assessment can be facilitated using all practical strategies to enhance understanding and communication including talking, sign language, visual aids or any other means.

The Mental Capacity Act Code of Practice (2007) provides a more detailed description of what the MCA (2005) means in day-to-day practice. The code or practice recommends an SLT be consulted to formally assess patients who have communication difficulties and to support the capacity assessment itself. They highlight the value of a multidisciplinary capacity assessment. Case study 1 is an example of where an SLT could have been involved much earlier to maximise long- term outcomes.

Individuals are often considered as potentially lacking capacity when they decide to follow a path that seems 'risky' or simply the opposite of that which the 'wise' health professional has recommended. Yet, as the MCA (2005) highlights, it is not our role to judge the decisions another person makes. In addition, the MCA Code of Practice (2007) emphasises that everyone has his or her own values, beliefs, preferences and attitudes. Our role is to support the individual to make decisions if they are able to do so, and protect them from harm should they not have capacity to make decisions. When a person makes a series of unwise choices, this can act as a flag to those around them to consider assessing capacity, but should not form the only basis for this justification.

Case Study 1

"The careful assessment of whether individuals have or lack capacity is essential to the protection of their rights" (BMA and The Law Society, 2004).

A young aphasic man was admitted to A&E with a medical condition. The medical team managed the condition but the man was left with ongoing issues for which further surgery was recommended. This decision was discussed with the individual's father without the individual himself being fully involved (i.e. without consulting any SLT or using any communication aids). His father was not appointed as his power of attorney for welfare decisions, but consented to the surgery, and the surgery was deemed 'successful'. An SLT saw the young man following the surgery and it was at this time that he was able to raise his concerns about the surgery. The young man felt distressed that he did not understand what had happened and what this meant for his future. The SLT used verbal, written and drawn diagrams over a number of sessions to explain the medical issue he had experienced and the consequent surgery, as well as addressing his future physical health needs by attending medical appointments as an advocate. Having discussed this information, the young man demonstrated he was able to understand, retain and weigh up this information as well as communicate his decision. He demonstrated capacity to make the decision and approved of the decisions that had been made. It is unfortunate that the A&E team had assumed that this gentleman lacked capacity. Consequently, the SLT provided a written document in his medical record addressing his capacity and communication needs. The document highlighted that, should future decisions need to be made regarding his medical needs, the young man may be able to demonstrate decision-making capacity, should appropriate supports and a SLT be consulted.

It can be easy for health professionals to assume that someone who is struggling to articulate their decision lacks capacity. Thus, a decision they communicate that seems to be at odds with our opinion is additional evidence of their lack of capacity. This highlights the need for a full and proper assessment of capacity, and the use of the multidisciplinary team to support this process. The individual may simply be lacking the information to make a full and proper decision, in which case it can be an advantage for the person to be seen on a number of occasions over a period of time in order to fully appreciate all the information. The MCA Code of Practice (2007) emphasises that complex issues may require fuller assessments, for example by different experts within the team including psychologists, SLTs and medical staff.

Case Study 2

"Capacity is the pivotal issue in balancing the right to autonomy in decision making and the right to protection from harm" (BMA and The Law Society, 2004).

Mr Y is admitted to hospital with a stroke. He presents with ongoing dysphagia almost a year following his stroke. He remains in hospital undergoing rehabilitation for the remaining disabilities that include mobility, speech and various physical limitations. He has demonstrated no improvements in his swallowing and remains on a pureed diet with syrup thick fluids. He has requested that he be upgraded to a normal diet. He has undergone video-fluoroscopy X-rays that have been used to show him his on-going risks of choking and aspiration. He demonstrates a good understanding of the consequences of choking and aspiration, and has requested a 'do not resuscitate' order should he choke. His family feel that this type of request is consistent with his previous and current priorities around enjoying his food above all else. Mr Y demonstrates a good understanding of the possibility that his swallow could perhaps improve in the future at some point, but he continues to express a preference to eat normal foods against speech and language therapy advice. He has been assessed by the team (including the neuro and clinical psychologist and medical team) to demonstrate a good understanding of the decision, to retain information, to weigh this information appropriately and communicate his preferences. He does not present with any mood disorders. It was decided that Mr Y had the capacity to decide not to follow the recommendations even though it was perceived to be an unwise decision by the treating team.

Case study 2 emphasises the value of using the multidisciplinary team in supporting someone to make their own capacitous decision.

It can be challenging for health professionals to support people in their 'unwise decisions' but it is our role to advocate for our patients. It is not uncommon for conflicts to be led by National Health Service (NHS) targets and financial pressures. At times, advocating for our patients can be at odds with issues such as bed space and care costs. What a health professional may assume is least restrictive, such as getting out of hospital quickly, for that individual may not be their top priority (as illustrated in Case study 3).

The MCA Code of Practice (2007) highlights that "It is important to *explore* ways that would be less restrictive or allow the most freedom for a person who lacks capacity to make the decision in question" (p. 27). This means that we need to consider options other than those that may be at the forefront of our minds, when considering best interests. Case study 3 demonstrates how we can consider a patient's situation in their best interests.

Case Study 3

Mrs H presents to hospital with a medical history of MS, a recent chest infection and severe dysphagia. She is recommended to commence non-oral feeding and a naso-gastric tube is inserted. The medical team feels she is recovering slowly from her chest infection and dysphagia. They advocate that she consider a percutaneous endoscopic gastrostomy (PEG) tube so that she can be discharged home more promptly. The patient's husband informs the SLT that his wife has previously experienced an episode of dysphagia and returned to a normal diet in due course; he is reluctant to consider a PEG tube as he reports that she would have preferred not to have a PEG inserted. Mrs H is unable to engage in any verbal or nonverbal discussion surrounding this issue, and has been assessed as lacking capacity. In a best-interests meeting, the SLT recommends that the lady has already made some gains in her swallowing and may be able to continue to recover. It is decided that the least restrictive options for this lady is to remain on the ward and await any further improvements in her swallowing before considering whether to proceed with a PEG tube insertion.

Case Study 4

A gentleman who had sustained a brain injury was admitted to a rehabilitation ward. He stated to the team that, although he found the therapies and ward environment stimulating, he did not wish to remain on the ward and preferred to return home. Prior to the injury, this gentleman had been living at home with his mother. He had been a very successful businessman, had married and had two children. However, after his wife left him due to his excessive alcohol usage, he continued to drink and lost his business after going into debt. He moved in with his mother where he continued drinking and had consequently suffered a brain injury when he fell down a staircase whilst under the influence of alcohol. At his previous facility, he had often gone out and returned to the ward after drinking heavily. He had also experienced a number of seizures, one with almost life-threatening consequences. On his admission to the ward, this gentleman presented well, he was polite and able to understand questions in conversation and explain clearly that he wished to return home. Yet on communication and neuropsychology assessment it was found that he demonstrated difficulties in memory, reasoning and judgement. He also denied that his seizures could be associated with his alcohol usage and stated that he planned to continue drinking. On assessing his decision-making capacity in relation to returning home and using alcohol, the treating team felt that he could not retain nor appropriately weigh up the issues relating to the risks to his own health. It was consequently decided that he lacked the capacity to make this decision. A best interests meeting was held with his mother and an Independent Mental Capacity Advocate (IMCA) present. The team agreed that it was in his best interests at this stage to remain on the ward and engage in therapies, which he was fully engaging in and, furthermore, making gains in.

Persons who lack capacity

Assessing someone's capacity may not always be so straightforward. As stated previously, there must be evidence that the individual has 'a disturbance in the functioning of the mind or brain'. A person who presents with dysarthria may be assumed to have a disturbance of the functioning of their mind or brain, they may seem drunk or be assumed to lack the intellectual skills to make decisions. An older adult may be assumed to lack capacity simply because of society's perception around their age and gender. Equally, an individual may be assumed to have capacity if they present themselves well, are articulate and physically able.

The process of balancing probabilities is more complex than this and requires expertise and sensitivity to the issues in question. An SLT is an expert in assessing a person's ability to communicate and differentiating between cognitive and communication skills that could impact on the decision in question. Case study 4 illustrates the various issues that a specialist team may need to discuss and consider in this process. Balancing these issues needs to done carefully, being mindful of the impact on the individual, their future engagement and those around them. Case study 4 highlights that assessing capacity could affect therapeutic relationships, and this in turn needs to be weighed up by the treating team. It may not always be most appropriate for the SLT, or their immediate family members, to advocate for the person. These issues around roles and advocates are further discussed in Chapter 7.

Inability to make decisions

Having proven that an individual has a disturbance of the functioning of the brain or mind, the assessment may proceed. The MCA (2005) provides a clear definition to guide an assessment of decision-making comprising four specific questions to consider. These four areas should be addressed directly during the assessment considering the following details. The MCA Code of Practice (2007) makes specific recommendations with regard to these areas. Case study 5 illustrates how each area may be considered in an individual with communication difficulties.

(a) Understanding the information

The person must be provided with information before the assessment of their understanding is commenced. Without the information the person will not be able to demonstrate an appropriate understanding. The Code of Practice (2007) recommends this cover:

- the nature of the decision;
- the reason why the decision is needed; and
- the likely effects of deciding one way or another, or making no decision at all.

This information should be presented in an appropriate way using simple language, visual aids or any other means. It should be translated into the appropriate language required should that individual not speak an adequate level of English. Information may be presented verbally over a number of occasions; it may be that the information needs to be translated to an aphasia-friendly format. Equally, the information may need to be presented visually in pictorial format.

Case Study 5: Understanding

A lady is admitted to a rehabilitation ward following her third stroke. She presents with aphasia, dysarthria and a number of physical limitations. She also presents with some cognitive difficulties. This lady has previously had a successful cataract operation and requires another. Her better eye has unfortunately been affected by the stroke and she has limited vision in this eye too. The opthalmology consultant recommends a cataract operation but is concerned that she does not understand the recommendations and the risks. She attends the appointment with the SLT who is able to take away the written information. They discuss the content of the information leaflet, the SLT reads the leaflet aloud and explains any key words the patient feels are unclear. On returning to the ophthalmology consultant a fortnight later, she is able to demonstrate her understanding of the procedure by explaining what has been read to her.

(b) Retaining information

To retain that information, a person must be able to hold the information long enough in their minds to make an effective decision (this may mean they only need to retain information for the course of the assessment session). If a person demonstrates difficulties retaining information this does not automatically mean they lack capacity. Assessments of capacity may be conducted over a number of occasions to ensure consistency in their decision-making. The MCA Code of Practice (2007) suggests that a person may use aids to support their memory quite effectively, including notebooks, diaries, signage or posters, voice or video recordings.

Case Study 5 (cont): Retaining information

The lady is able to demonstrate that she can retain information and relevant concerns about the risks that she wishes to address with the consultant between chatting to the SLT and the next appointment with the doctor. Although the SLT had planned to prompt her with a key word this is not required. The lady is spontaneously able to recall aspects of her previous operation and apply them to this scenario. She demonstrates an ability to retain information within the discussion, reporting back to the consultant that she is satisfied with his answers, which she can repeat back to us, before making her decision to consent to the process.

(c) Using or weighing up information

To demonstrate capacity, an individual must be able to use or weigh up information as part of the process of arriving at a decision. Individuals may understand information they have been given, but due to a disturbance in their brain or mind they may not be able to consider the benefits or risks of the information provided. They may make decisions impulsively if they have had a brain injury, or because beliefs relating to their mental health diagnosis prevent them from weighing information up effectively. The MCA Code of Practice (2007) provides the example of an individual with anorexia nervosa who may understand the information about the consequences of not eating but their underlying compulsions may be too significant to ignore.

Case Study 5 (cont): Using information

The lady generates a list of questions related to the procedure and the risks of a cataract operation that she asks the ophthalmology consultant at the next appointment with the support of the SLT. These include questions about the likelihood of the listed 'risks' occurring to her, the aftercare requirements and how these will interact with her other medical issues. This demonstrates a good ability to integrate and consider information relevant to the decision

(d) Communicating a decision

An individual needs to demonstrate their ability to communicate their decision using all practical and appropriate methods and aids to support this, whether by talking, using sign language or any other aids. The Code of Practice (2007) highlights that there may be some situations where a person cannot communicate, for example if they are in a coma, or unconscious. People with rare conditions such as Locked-in Syndrome can still use eye movements, e-Tran boards, and other low or high technology aids to communicate their preferences. In these cases, the former three domains of the capacity assessment must also be satisfied to confirm the individual actually has capacity.

Case Study 5 (cont): Communicating a decision

The lady is able to plan her questions for the consultant in the sessions with the SLT. The SLT documents the questions and informs the consultant that the patient has a series of questions, when the lady asks the questions. The lady is not always intelligible but as a familiar listener the SLT is able to clarify what the consultant does not understand when the individual is speaking to him.

Both the SLT and the Consultant Ophthalmologist agreed that she had capacity to make the decision and the surgery went ahead the next week. The SLT did not attend the surgery but the Consultant requested advice on the type of language to use to re-check her capacity at the time of the surgery.

Conclusions

The core ethical principles of health care decision-making include: respect for autonomy; supporting patients to self-determine their future, and beneficence; protecting from harm. It was not until the latter half of the 20th century that we, as a society, became more interested in how this works for our loved ones. It is also worth flagging that the heightened emphasis on self-determination is largely a western phenomenon and not universally shared. Thus, assessing decision-making capacity is a somewhat novel concept for health professionals, but one in which we are becoming more literate.

The MCA (2005) and the accompanying Code of Practice (2007) provide a detailed definition of mental capacity and how to manage the issues surrounding capacity for health professionals. Communication is the key to assessing decision-making capacity, and SLTs should be involved in these types of assessments when people have difficulties in any aspect of communication, or when the decision is directly related to dysphagia. The case studies described in this chapter endeavour to illustrate our role. The next chapter will develop this further with more case studies illustrating other relevant sections of the MCA (2005).

References

British Medical Association and The Law Society (2004) *Mental Capacity: Guidance for doctors and lawyers*, 2nd ed. London, BMJ Books.

Bronte, Charlotte (1847) *Jane Eyre*. London, Smith, Elder & Co.

Lawton-Smith, S. & McCulloch, A. A brief history of specialist mental health services. (Viewed online April 2015) Mental Health Foundation. http://www.mentalhealth.org.uk/content/assets/pdf/publications/starting-today-background-paper-1.pdf

Mental Capacity Act 2005:

http://www.legislation.gov.uk/ukpga/2005/9/pdfs/ukpga_20050009_en.pdfThe Mental Health Act 2005

Mental Capacity Act 2005 Code of Practice (2007): http://www.legislation.gov.uk/ukpga/2005/9/pdfs/ukpgacop_20050009_en.pdf

Mental Health Act 1959: http://www.legislation.gov.uk/ukpga/1959/72/pdfs/ukpga_19590072_en.pdf

Mentalhealthcare.org.uk website advice (viewed January 2015) http://www.mentalhealthcare.org.uk/mental_health_act

Mental Health Act 1983: An outline guide. A useful summary of the Act from 'Mind', including updated material to take account of the Mental Health Act 2007. http://www.mind.org.uk/media/7505/the-mind-guide-to-the-mental-health-act-1983-2012.pdf

Mental Health Act 2007 (viewed online January 2015) http://www.legislation.gov.uk/ukpga/2007/12/contents

Moncreiff, J. (2003) The politics of a new Mental Health Act. *The British Journal of Psychiatry*, 183: 8–9. DOI: 10.1192/bjp.183.1.8

The National Archives Website (viewed January 2015) http://www.nationalarchives.gov.uk/records/research-guides/mental-health.htm

Re Airedale National Health Service Trust v Bland, (1993) 1 All ER 821.

Re F [2000] EWCA Civ. 192 (Butler-Sloss LJ, Thorpe LJ, Sedley LJ)

Re Hinde, ex parte Whitbread [1816] 2 Mer 99 (Lord Eldon).

Re L (WJG) [1966] Ch 135 (Cross J)

Re SL (Adult Patient) (Medical Treatment) [2001] Fam. 15 (Butler-Sloss, Thorpe and Mance LJ).

Sense Website (viewed September 2015) https://www.sense.org.uk/content/law-and-mental-capacity

Szerletics, A. (2012) Best interests decision-making under the Mental Capacity Act. (Viewed January 2015) http://autonomy.essex.ac.uk/best-interests-decision-making-under-the-mental-capacity-act

The Adults with Incapacity (Scotland) Act (2000): http://www.legislation.gov.uk/asp/2000/4/contents

3 Demystifying the Mental Capacity Act:

Making Best Interests Decisions, Lasting Power of Attorney and Deputy roles, Independent Mental Capacity Advocates and Deprivation of Liberty Safeguards

Anna Volkmer

Introduction

People who lack capacity are vulnerable to the risks of impaired decision-making. Whilst clinicians need to ensure that capable patients have the opportunity to make treatment decisions they also need to ensure that those who are lacking decision-making capacity are protected. This is where it is important to understand the processes of a 'best interests decision' and the role of proxy decision-makers such as Lasting Power of Attorneys (LPAs) and Deputies compared to Advocates.

The media and public interest in proxy decision-making and advance decisions has increased. Healthy people are increasingly making advance decisions and nominating decision-makers while they have capacity, with the view that they are preparing for when they may not. In reality, there are very few people who have actually nominated these roles to the people they love. Consequently, people who have lost capacity may need Deputies to be appointed to support them in their day-to-day affairs.

The Mental Capacity Act (MCA, 2005) seeks to provide guidance on all these areas, including the aforementioned best interest decisions, LPA and Independent Mental Capacity Advocates (IMCAs). The MCA complements other acts such as the Mental Health Act 1983. An individual may be detained, or 'sectioned' as it is informally known, for assessment, treatment or care under the Mental Health Act if they have a mental disorder that causes risk to themselves or others. Individuals who are detained under the Mental Health Act do not necessarily lack capacity. Other individuals may not need to be detained in this way, but may lack capacity and may be prevented from leaving a facility such as a residential facility as they are considered vulnerable adults. In these cases, it may be considered that these individuals are being deprived of their liberties. The Deprivation of Liberty Safeguards (DoLS) section of the MCA is currently under review, but it has aimed to provide guidance and support in these cases.

As in the previous chapter, this chapter will shed more light on these aspects of the MCA (2005) using case studies relevant to speech and language therapists (SLTs).

Making best interests decisions

If a person lacks capacity to make decisions, a decision may need to be made for them. This is called making a 'best interests decision'. It is important that best interests decisions are only made if the person's capacity has been appropriately assessed and it has been shown that the individual lacks capacity. Otherwise, the person carrying out the consequent act or omission (i.e. medical treatment or lack thereof) may risk incurring liability for that act. In case study 1 in Chapter 2, this practice was not observed and, indeed, if it were to happen in real life the health professionals involved could be at risk of future litigation.

Where possible, a decision should be postponed. For example, a less urgent medical or financial decision might be postponed until a person is no longer under the influence of drugs or alcohol or until they regain consciousness and potentially regain their capacity. However, a life and limb decision (a decision related to the continued existence or serious injury of the person in question), may need to be made immediately on their behalf, i.e. out of necessity in their best interests.

Some individuals may not be expected to regain capacity, thus some decisions cannot or should not be delayed. For example, an adult with dementia may not be expected to regain capacity to make a decision about their living circumstances. The MCA (2005) section 4 (4) states that when making best interest decisions "as far as reasonably practicable, permit and encourage the person to participate, or to improve his ability to participate, as fully as possible in any act done for him and any decision affecting him". In these situations it may be the SLT's role to engage the person with communication difficulties in a discussion about their preferences using the appropriate communication techniques and aids. These supports may include tools such as Talking Mats© (see Figure 5.1; Murphy et al., 2010) or the Supporting Adults with Communication Impairment to make Decisions resource (see Figure 5.2; Allen and Bryer, 2014) that can support people with communication difficulties in contributing to decision-making (see case study 1 below).

Communicating can be challenging, and it is important to be sure that a vulnerable person is not influenced or persuaded by another person's views. Using leading questions may be considered as skewing a person's responses by providing them with the desired outcomes or ideas. Many 'patients' simply want to give the answers they feel that others want from them, rather than those that they believe. Equally, vulnerable (and suggestible) adults may easily be influenced by other external factors such as their peers. Gathering information and evidence to understand a person's belief system helps the treating team to make a balanced best interest decision.

But who does the decision-making? If an LPA has been nominated and registered, or a Deputy has been appointed under a court order, they will be the decision-maker for decisions within the scope of their authority. Should there not be a nominated LPA or Deputy, the MCA Code of Practice (2007) emphasises that for most day-to-day decisions, the decision-maker will be "the carer most directly involved with the person at the time". This may be the family member, nurse or paid carer. Where the decision involves the provision of medical treatment, the doctor or other member of healthcare staff, including the SLT, responsible for carrying out the particular treatment or procedure will act as the decision-maker. Often these types of decisions will be made jointly, by a group of people, for example the multidisciplinary team. An SLT may well be the primary decision-maker when, for example, judging whether it is in the person's best interests to be involved in the assessment or treatment session they are delivering (see case study 5). Equally, SLTs may form part of the team involved in making a more significant decision related to health, care or finances (see case studies 1 and 2 in this chapter).

Case Study 1

Mr M has a diagnosis of moderate Lewy Body dementia. He is an inpatient in a nursing home and has been referred for an assessment of his swallow function by the nursing staff. They report he has recently been choking on foods and are concerned about his risk of choking again. He is mobile and often wanders around the unit. When introduced to the SLT, Mr M presents with evident cognitive difficulties and is not orientated to the situation; he believes he is on a cruise ship and the SLT is a member of the crew. He is unable to understand what the SLT explains about the referral, he cannot retain any details nor is he able to use the advice given; he evidently lacks capacity. However, he is agreeable to spending time with the therapist and is compliant with assessment. In view of the concerns of the nursing staff the SLT decides that it is in Mr M's best interests to continue with the assessment process. However, before Mr M has had anything to eat or drink he spots his relatives entering the unit. They notice a professional is present and turn to leave. He becomes quite distressed and starts shouting to them and tries to stand up to walk over to them. Mr M remains distressed and agitated for the next five minutes and declines to eat or drink. The SLT decides that it is in his best interests to cease the session in order to invite his family into the room and complete the assessment. The SLT invites the family to sit with them for some food and drinks and is able to complete her assessment.

The MCA (2005) states that people making the decisions must consider, "so far as is reasonably ascertainable–

1. the person's past and present wishes and feelings (and, in particular, any relevant written statement made by him when he had capacity),

2. the beliefs and values that would be likely to influence his decision if he had capacity, and

3. the other factors that he would be likely to consider if he were able to do so" (Section 4, 6).

Establishing a person's preference or wishes may not always be as straightforward as using a picture-led communication tool. Many individuals cannot express their wishes and feelings in words but may express themselves through their behaviour, for example lashing out or verbal abuse when treatment is being offered or provided. An SLT may be asked to advise the treating team or decision-maker on how best to interpret an individual's communication attempts and behaviours. Identifying alternative methods of communication can be challenging for health professionals who are not communication experts.

A small minority of people have written advance directives which will negate the need to have a best interests meeting. However, there may be other sources of information that can be used in making a best interests decision. Some people may have recorded their wishes and beliefs on paper, video or audio-recordings in an attempt to support future decision-making about their care. These are not legal documents but may be useful tools to gain an insight to people's past wishes and beliefs. More evidence can be sought from, for example, their religious, political and cultural background and beliefs as well as their past behaviours and habits. This information can often be provided by those closest to them (see Case study 2).

Case Study 2

Mrs R has had aphasia following a stroke some time ago. She has recently also been diagnosed with dementia. Her husband was appointed as her enduring power of attorney for financial decisions following the stroke. He has been considering selling their jointly-owned home as they have both been struggling with the stairs, and Mrs R has recently fallen on the stairs. He feels anxious about the impact that this decision could have on his wife, as she loves their home, but they have no finances to modify the home. He is keen to buy a small bungalow closer to their children (a son and daughter who both live a couple of hours away). He speaks to an SLT about his concerns and they jointly used the Talking Mats© tool over a series of sessions with Mrs R. During these sessions the SLT familiarises Mrs R with pictures of their daily activities, images of their home, different rooms in the house and other types of homes. She also provides images of the area they live in and the areas where their children live. Mrs R is then asked to rate what is difficult or easy about living in their home. She is unable to identify what is easy or hard, stating everything is fine. When asked to rate where she would like to live, as her husband predicted she states that she does not wish to move,. Mrs R is then asked what could be changed about their home.

She states that she would like to add more rooms so her daughter, and particularly her grandchildren, could stay with them regularly. Mr R then feels more able proceed in applying to the Court of Protection with his decision to sell their home. He feels the information that he and the SLT have gathered will support him in considering his wife preferences in his decision-making. It is agreed that although Mrs R lacks capacity to make this decision she has expressed a preference to see her daughter and grandchildren more, which guides Mr R in searching for a property near his daughter. The SLT documents these events and writes a report to Mrs R's GP.

Ensuring that a decision is in the best interests of an individual includes considering not just their physical welfare (health, care needs and consistency) but also of their emotional needs (importance of relationships and sense of belonging). The MCA (2005) highlights that part of the process of making an appropriate best interests decision should include discussions with family who may be able to shed light on the person's wishes, beliefs and preferences. The people caring for the person on a daily basis may know the person well and thus may know how they are likely to cope with the consequences. When making decisions in someone's best interests it is not always possible or practical to ensure you have considered all aspects of the decision and how they would and could impact upon the person. The MCA (2005) defines the most relevant issues or circumstances that need to be considered as those (section 4,11):

> "(a) of which the person making the determination is aware, and
>
> (b) which it would be reasonable to regard as relevant."

In case study 2, Mr R and the SLT needed to consider the benefits to Mrs R, in terms of both her physical, financial and emotional welfare as well as the similar needs of her husband, Mr R. This included whether living somewhere else would make things easier for both parties concerned, whether things might change in the future and whether Mrs R could stay safer 'in her home' for longer if the environment were better set up for her physical and mental needs.

At times, making a best interests decision can be very difficult for us as health professionals. Our recommendations as SLTs may reduce the risk of our clients choking or having a chest infection but, equally, may significantly reduce a person's perceived quality of life. This often arises when discussing dysphagia-related recommendations, and as SLTs it is important for us to be able to accept an individual's wishes even if we feel this is an unwise decision (see case study 3). People may hold values or beliefs that have guided them in this decision-making, and these may be contrary to our own. Ethically, as therapists we must accept an individual's right to make these types of decisions, and come to terms with this. Supporting a decision which we feel is 'unwise' is often easier said than done. The MCA (2007) Code of Practice acknowledges this dilemma and recommends that health professionals should raise this issue with the patient where possible, although this will often not be possible where this is made as a best interests decision. The MCA Code of Practice (2007) recommends a clinician should endeavour to continue to support the patient but, if necessary, consider moving the care of the individual to another professional, without abandoning them.

Roles of Lasting Power of Attorney and Deputy

Sometimes an individual may wish to nominate another person to make decisions for them when they are no longer able to do so. A Lasting Power of Attorney (LPA) is given by a person (who is over 18 years of age) when they still retain decision-making capacity and comes into power only when they no longer have capacity. This is defined by the MCA (2005) as:

> "a power of attorney under which the donor ("P") confers on the donee (or donees) authority to make decisions about all or any of the following—
>
> (a) P's personal welfare or specified matters concerning P's personal welfare, and
>
> (b) P's property and affairs or specified matters concerning P's property and affairs,
>
> and which includes authority to make such decisions in circumstances where P no longer has capacity" (Section 9,1).

More than one person may be nominated to hold an LPA. Once given an LPA, the donee cannot transfer their role to others or appoint a successor. Consequently, the MCA (2005) lays out that if there is more than one appointed attorney (LPA), the donor should decide in advance if he or she would like those people to make all their decisions jointly (together) or whether one person can make a decision on their own (i.e. jointly or severally). For example, a parent prefers their three children to jointly hold the role of LPA. One of these children lives further away, thus it may be convenient for decisions to be made by these children individually (i.e. severally).

Case Study 3

Mr M has Parkinson's disease and lives at home with his wife who provides all his care. He has been assessed at home and diagnosed with a worsened dysphagia, and the SLT recommends that he should be on thickened drinks and a modified diet. Mr M has had Parkinson's disease for some time and has developed significant cognitive difficulties, which means he does not have the capacity to make a decision related to this issue. Mrs M is particularly concerned as she finds that Mr M has become very picky, and will only eat specific foods from a narrow range of options such as ham sandwiches, toast, pies, roast dinners and fish and chips. Mrs M has tried cooking foods such a soups, stews and softer foods as per the recommendations given by a previous SLT, but her husband would become distressed, decline foods and lose weight. Mrs M explains that her husband had been a chef in a local traditional English restaurant and had always enjoyed his food. She feels that he would never have wanted to modify his foods or drinks in such a way as recommended. She feels strongly that he would wish to continue eating and drinking the things he enjoyed even with the risks of choking or chest infections. Mrs M demonstrates a good understanding of the risks of aspiration and choking, and continues to insist on what she feels are her husband's preferences even following a videofluoroscopy that confirms the recommendations. Had he written an advance directive stating these wishes it would be clear which recommendations would be in his best interests. Had he nominated his wife the role of LPA for health and welfare decisions, similarly it would be clear that she would have been legally able to advocate for his best interests with this position. A discussion is held between the GP, the dietitian and SLT. They agree that enforcing the recommendations would not be in Mr M's emotional or physical best interests as they do not wish him to lose weight, nor wish to remove him from his wife's care as in all other matters she has followed health professionals' advice. It is agreed his wife is advocating appropriately for her husband's wishes, and that the team should allow her to continue providing her husband with the foods she feels he will eat. Finally, it is agreed that the SLT and dietitian will continue to provide support to Mr and Mrs M to problem solve any issues that arise.

In order to donate the role of LPA, a written document must be set in the statutory format as required by the current regulations. The document must include specific information detailing the type of attorney (LPA) being donated: financial or welfare. Both the donor and donee must be named and have signed the document and a third party must certify the document. An LPA must be registered with the Office of the Public Guardian before it can be used. However, once the LPA is registered, the attorney is able to make all decisions about the donor's property and affairs even if the donor still has capacity to make the decisions for themselves and this will continue to apply when the donor no longer has capacity. This does not apply to personal welfare decisions.

Holding the role of LPA for personal welfare decisions means the attorney is able to "give or refuse consent to the carrying out or continuation of a treatment by a person providing health care for P" (section 25, 2). This means that had Mrs M in case study 3 held the position of LPA for health and welfare she would have been able to legitimately decline the treatment recommendation of the SLT on behalf of her husband.

It is important to note here that if a clinician believes that the person with power of attorney is not acting in the person's 'best interests' they may appeal to courts to review their position. These doubts may arise in instances where, for example, the LPA is using the person's finances for their own benefit or making decisions about health and welfare that could actively result in death or harm to the individual. The MCA states that the role of LPA "does not authorise the giving or refusing of consent to the carrying out or continuation of life-sustaining treatment, unless the instrument contains express provision to that effect" (section 11, 8). Examples of this include the withdrawal of artificial feeding (percutaneous endoscopic gastronomy tubes), or ventilation, both of which could not be refused by an LPA. Table 3.1 summarises the types of decisions that may be made by LPAs, both financial and welfare related.

It is not uncommon that a patient may lack capacity to make decisions related to their finances or complex medical decisions, and requires an LPA or

Table 3.1 Property, financial and welfare Lasting Power of Attorney (LPA) decisions may include the following examples (summarised from examples in the Code of Practice, 2007).

Property and financial LPAs might include decisions about:	Personal welfare LPAs might include decisions about:
Buying or selling property	Where the donor should live and who they should live with
Opening, closing or operating any bank, building society or other account	The donor's day-to-day care, including diet and dress
Giving access to the donor's financial information	Who the donor may have contact with
Claiming, receiving and using (on the donor's behalf) all benefits, pensions, allowances and rebates (unless the Department for Work and Pensions has already appointed someone and everyone is happy for this to continue)	Consenting to or refusing medical examination and treatment on the donor's behalf
Receiving any income, inheritance or other entitlement on behalf of the donor	Arrangements needed for the donor to be given medical, dental or optical treatment
Dealing with the donor's tax affairs	Assessments for and provision of community care services
Paying the donor's mortgage, rent and household expenses	Whether the donor should take part in social activities, leisure activities, education or training
Insuring, maintaining and repairing the donor's property	The donor's personal correspondence and papers
Investing the donor's savings	Rights of access to personal information about the donor
Making limited gifts on the donor's behalf	Complaints about the donor's care or treatment.
Paying for private medical care and residential care or nursing home fees	
Applying for any entitlement to funding for NHS care, social care or adaptations	
Using the donor's money to buy a vehicle or any equipment or other help they need	
Repaying interest and capital on any loan taken out by the donor	

Deputy to deal with this. Yet even if they lack decision-making capacity for these skills it should not be assumed that they do not have other decision-making abilities. Indeed, they may still have capacity to appoint the person they wish to help make these more complex decisions (Mitty & Fraber-Post, 2008). This should be separately assessed. As previously highlighted, capacity is decision-specific rather than global, and may fluctuate depending on clinical condition, medication or time of day. Should the patient lack the decision-making ability to appoint an attorney (LPA), they may still be able to express a preference for the assignment of a Deputy. Considering an individual's preferences around this role may enhance their ability to participate in decision-making and comply with the outcomes of decisions made on their behalf. Compliance and engagement can be a big challenge and should be considered in long-term decisions such as this.

Deputy

The MCA (2005) outlined the provision for a new specialist court called the Court of Protection. This replaced the previous Court of Protection, which only dealt with decisions about the property and financial affairs of people lacking capacity. The new Court of Protection deals with property and affairs and serious decisions affecting healthcare and personal welfare matters for people who lack capacity.

It is not practical for the court to make every decision for an individual who is unlikely to regain capacity. The Court of Protection can appoint a Deputy to make decisions for people who lack capacity to make those decisions or may remove a Deputy or attorney who acts inappropriately. Often the court will appoint a family member or someone who knows the person well as a Deputy (see case study 4). In some cases, the Court of Protection may decide to appoint someone independent if the person's needs are particularly complex (e.g. a professional Deputy; often a solicitor who specialises in this area of law).

If a Deputy is appointed there are still some situations where an application to the Court of Protection may be necessary. The Court of Protection tends only to get involved with particularly difficult decisions, or when there are disagreements. This includes decisions about the proposed withholding or withdrawal of artificial nutrition and hydration from patients in a permanent vegetative state. These will also include dealing with significant cash assets over a specified amount that remain after any debts have been paid or for selling a person's property.

Case Study 4

Mr J is a 53-year-old man who sustained a brain injury in a car accident. He is now in his 9th month following the injury and is planning to return home to his family, with his wife as his primary carer. Mr J had not previously organised an LPA and his wife has been looking after the family finances in an ad hoc fashion since the injury. The rehabilitation team is preparing Mr J for his discharge and identify that it is unlikely that he will regain his decision-making capacity for financial decisions. The SLT identifies that his aphasia has not improved all that much since his injury and he is unable to read bills or communicate with unfamiliar listeners easily. Together with the Occupational Therapist (OT), the SLT identifies that Mr J also presents with cognitive difficulties and, although he has managed small monies up to £10.00 in small shopping tasks, he cannot budget larger amounts, he cannot recall his pin number, nor is he able to consider the risks that could arise if he did not pay bills or check his accounts regularly. The team feel that his aphasia and language skills are unlikely to improve significantly in the near future to enable him to manage his finances. The SLT and OT have completed a formal assessment of decision-making capacity and have found he lacks capacity in managing his finances. This has been documented in the medical notes. The team has recommended that he would benefit from a Deputy to support him in managing his finances. Mrs J is keen to take on this role and Mr J is agreeable to this arrangement. The medical consultant completes the required paperwork for Mrs J to take to the family's solicitor to apply to the Court of Protection for Mrs J to be assigned as a Deputy in order to manage his finances.

Advance decision making

The MCA (2005) describes an advance decision as:

> "a decision made by a person ("P"), after he has reached 18 and when he has capacity to do so, that if—

(a) at a later time and in such circumstances as he may specify, a specified treatment is proposed to be carried out or continued by a person providing health care for him, and

(b) at that time he lacks capacity to consent to the carrying out or continuation of the treatment, the specified treatment is not to be carried out or continued." (section 24,1)

Advance decisions and advance directives are discussed in depth later in this book. This chapter emphasises the important role SLTs can have in empowering people to consider making advance decisions in order to have a voice throughout their care, particularly for people with progressive conditions. Advance directives could be considered not only a legal document, but also a communication aid for a time when a person is no longer able to communicate their wishes.

Independent Mental Capacity Advocates

The MCA (2005) has also provided a description of a new role: an Independent Mental Capacity Advocate (IMCA). This service should be available to individuals who lack decision-making capacity, are facing serious decisions and have nobody else to represent them or who could be consulted. The Office of the Public Guardian has produced a number of booklets outlining the roles of the IMCA and the type of serious decisions they may be involved with. These may include issues such as discharge from hospital to a new long-term residence that is different to their previous residence, e.g. moving into a nursing home or residential facility where they had previously been living at home independently, or deciding on a serious medical treatment such as whether to undergo an operation such as a hip replacement (see case study 5).

The MCA (2005) outlines the functions of the IMCA as follows:

"(a) providing support to the person whom he has been instructed to represent ("P") so that P may participate as fully as possible in any relevant decision;

(b) obtaining and evaluating relevant information;

(c) ascertaining what P's wishes and feelings would be likely to be, and the beliefs and values that would be likely to influence P, if he had capacity;

(d) ascertaining what alternative courses of action are available in relation to P;

(e) obtaining a further medical opinion where treatment is proposed and the advocate thinks that one should be obtained." (section 36, 2)

NHS employees involved with the person lacking capacity are responsible for referring an individual to an IMCA. As someone completely independent to the team making the decisions, the IMCA can then provide support for the person who lacks capacity. This will include coming to meetings and best interests discussions to represent or support the person, as well as raising questions or challenges in regard to the decision should they feel it is not in the person's best interests.

The MCA Code of Practice (2007) explains that in England the Secretary of State for Health delivers the IMCA service through local authorities, who work in partnership with NHS organisations. Local authorities have financial responsibility for the service. In Wales, the National Assembly for Wales delivers the service through local health boards who have financial responsibility for the service and work in partnership with local authority social services departments and other NHS organisations. The service is commissioned from independent organisations, usually advocacy organisations (Social Care Institute for Excellence SCIE website, viewed September 2015). Every NHS organisation should have a relationship with a local IMCA service. However, the SCIE website (2014) does publish a list of IMCA providers according to the relevant geographical areas, should you need to find one (http://www.scie.org.uk/publications/imca/files/imca_providers.pdf).

Once a referral has been made, the IMCA must gather information in order to decide how best to represent and support the person that they are helping. This should include speaking to the person they are representing, examining medical records, speaking to the professionals and anybody else who can provide information or is involved with the person. When considering a person's best interests they should endeavour to establish the views, wishes, feelings, beliefs and values of the person they are representing, in the same way as described previously in this chapter regarding best interests decisions. Finally, they should write a report to the NHS organisation responsible for the patient they are representing.

The Office of the Public Guardian highlights that the IMCA should try to communicate with the person who lacks capacity using any means possible, including verbally and nonverbally and might mean using pictures or photographs. The RCSLT considers that an IMCA should be supported by the SLT in these types of interactions (RCSLT Dementia Position Paper, 2014; RCSLT, Response to draft Mental Capacity Bill Northern Ireland, 2014). This may include training or simply written guidance. Training of staff such as IMCAs is further discussed in Chapter 8.

Deprivation of Liberty Safeguards (DoLS)

If a person is admitted to hospital or placed in accommodation such as a nursing home or residential home they will need to consent to their admission. Should the individual in question lack the decision-making capacity to consent to this, and have no appointed attorney dealing with health and welfare who could give consent, then it will be considered that this person is being deprived of their liberty. There are conditions where this will not be the case, for example if someone has been detained under the Mental Health Act. The Deprivation of Liberty Safeguards (DoLS) aim to ensure that these individuals are cared for in a way that does not inappropriately or excessively restrict their liberties, when it is in their best interests and there are no other options available.

A recent definition of deprivation of liberty from two recent cases in the Supreme Court, "P v Cheshire West and Chester Council and another" and "P and Q v Surrey County Council", summarised by the Department of Health (2014) describes this as when: "the person is under continuous supervision and control and is not free to leave, and the person lacks capacity to consent to these arrangements" (p. 2). This suggests that any patients on a locked ward or unit who lacks capacity to consent to their admission should be considered under the DoLS and must be appropriately authorised. This will capture many patients with dementia or cognitive difficulties, who may or may not also be physically dependent on the staff around them.

The MCA (2005) emphasises that all options need to have been considered to provide care in the least possible restrictive manner. If these options have been explored, then a DoLS must be applied for and authorised in accordance with one of the following legal regimes: a deprivation of liberty authorisation or Court of Protection order under the DoLS in the Mental Capacity Act 2005, or (if applicable) under the Mental Health Act 1983 (Department of Health, 2014; Keene et al., 2014).

In some situations, being placed in hospital or in a residential or nursing home setting may be depriving an individual of their liberties. Even if this is in the person's best interests there may be no protection from liability unless the Court of Protection has deemed it in the person's best interests and have granted an order to this effect. In order to do this, the nursing home or NHS trust should apply for authorisation to the supervisory body (in England, the local authority). In Wales, this may be the local health board or the local authority. This should be done before or once the individual is admitted to hospital. If the person is in a supported living arrangement organised by the local authority the Court of Protection must authorise the deprivation of liberty. At this point, the supervisory body must assess the individual within 21 days, to establish whether they qualify for authorisation. This will include assessing their mental health, mental capacity, best interests and eligibility. Two assessors, a best interests assessor and a mental health assessor, appointed by the supervisory body, should complete this assessment. If all the conditions have been met the body will grant an authorisation, although they may ask for modifications to the individual's restrictions. This authorisation can remain valid for 12 months but must be regularly checked and removed when not required. In addition, the person's representative should be updated with information about their care on a regular basis. A review assessment may be triggered if there is a change in circumstance or it is not being managed in the least restrictive way.

It can be difficult to differentiate between restricting and depriving someone of their liberties; indeed, one large restriction could be considered a deprivation. There have been numerous examples of this issue being tested in case law, in the European Court of Human Rights and the UK. These have concluded that there are many situations as well as admission to hospital or a residential facility that can deprive someone of their liberties, including:

- physical restraint;

- medication being given against someone's will;

- staff being in control of someone's care or movements over a long period; and

- staff deciding issues such as visitors, treatment and assessments, discharge destination, access to friends and family.

These descriptions could include a number of patients whom SLTs may be treating. Any individual who is physically impaired, suffering from a stroke, brain injury or progressive neurological disease, could be deprived of their liberties in hospital or at home. As SLTs, we may be instrumental in the process of safeguarding an individual's liberties. This may include supporting staff to assess an individual's capacity to consent to their admission or flagging the need to apply for a DoLS assessment. Indeed Keene et al. (2014) emphasise that, even if an individual is living in their own home with their families but are being physically restrained from leaving should they attempt to, this could be considered a restriction. If any situation ever concerns you, it is important to speak to the treating team or your senior colleagues. You can also consult your Trust's MCA or DoLS representative or the Trust's legal team.

However, many medical professionals and health commentators highlight that "we currently have a confusing combination of two laws that might apply" (Ashby et al., 2015, p. 1), in reference to the MCA (2005) and the current Mental Health Act. It seems that protecting an individual from harm whilst respecting their liberties is a complex issue across many health settings. At the time of writing, the DoLS legislation is under review. Indeed, it continues to develop in case law as judges refine the interpretation of legal provisions. Keeping up with these changes is a challenge and will continue to be so. That said, this shouldn't discourage teams from discussing their concerns. Ultimately, if an action has been taken because it was considered in the person's best interests this can be considered the most ethical course of action. Unfortunately, ethics and law do not always keep up with one another and this in itself can be a challenge for health professionals.

Conclusions

The MCA (2005) does not just address the principles of assessing decision-making capacity, it also attempts to provide for the issues surrounding people who may lack capacity or may at some point in the future lack capacity. This includes making best interests decisions, appointing LPAs, Deputys and writing advance directives as well as the complex and grey area of DoLS. These are all areas that SLTs can and should be involved with. There will be specific times when we, as swallowing or communication experts, will be central to this process, for example, where a specific best interests decision may need to be made in relation to swallowing or where we are supporting people with communication difficulties to express their preferences or plan for their future.

These are not new issues to us as a discipline. SLTs are often one of the strongest advocates of making decisions which consider all aspects of a patient's 'best interests', for example, when considering taste for pleasure options for a person who is unsafe on all consistencies. We have long petitioned for our patients to have 'a voice' to assert their opinions and beliefs. Developing tools and documents, such as communication aids and life books, which enable a person with communication difficulties to express valuable information and preferences, is all part of this. Training families and caregivers to communicate with people with aphasia and dementia is also part of this. As previously emphasised, the MCA (2005) can be seen as a platform for SLTs to continue advocating for the needs of our patients. This will be further explored in the next chapters, which consider in more detail the process of assessment of decision-making capacity, the research evidence behind this and the type of training and advice we may be able to provide.

A word of warning, however: there will always be capable patients from cultures who do not value purely autonomous decisions and who may prefer to trust others in planning their care. In the same way that people with capacity have the right to make unwise decisions, they also have every right to delegate to a willing and able decision-maker.

Finally, if you are ever in any doubt about an individual patient and their needs, I would encourage you to speak to your colleagues and ultimately the MCA representative or your legal department within your organisation. These individuals have been appointed to discuss and assist clinicians in managing these types of issues.

References

Allen, J. & Bryer, H. (2014) *Supporting Adults with Communication Impairment to make Decisions*. UK, Blacksheep Press.

Ashby, G.A., Griffin, C. & Agrawal, N. (2015) Brain injury and deprivation of liberty on neurosciences wards: 'A gilded cage is still a cage'. *Practical Neurology*, 15(5): 361–368.

Department of Health Website (2014) Deprivation of Liberty Safeguards (DoLS) Judgment of the Supreme Court. P v Cheshire West and Chester Council and another P and Q v Surrey County Council. https://www.gov.uk/government/uploads/system/uploads/attachment_data/file/300106/DH_Note_re_Supreme_Court_DoLS_Judgment.pdf

Keene, A.R., Butler-Cole, V., Allen, N. & Bicarregui, A. (2014) Mental Capacity Law Guidance Note: Deprivation of Liberty after Cheshire West: Key questions for social workers and medical practitioners. Thirty Nine Essex Street Website (viewed September 2015) http://www.39essex.com/docs/newsletters/deprivation_of_liberty_after_cheshire_west_-_a_guide_for_front-line_staff.pdf

Mental Capacity Act 2005: http://www.legislation.gov.uk/ukpga/2005/9/pdfs/ukpga_20050009_en.pdfThe Mental Health Act 2005

Mental Capacity Act 2005 Code of Practice (2007): http://www.legislation.gov.uk/ukpga/2005/9/pdfs/ukpgacop_20050009_en.pdf

Mental Health Act 1983: An outline guide. A useful summary of the Act from 'Mind', including updated material to take account of the Mental Health Act 2007 http://www.mind.org.uk/media/7505/the-mind-guide-to-the-mental-health-act-1983-2012.pdf

Mitty, E. & Fraber-Post, L.(2008) Health care decision making. In: E. Capezuti, S. Zwicker, M. Mezey, T. Fulmer, D. Gray-Miceli & M. Kluger, *Evidence-Based Geriatric Nursing Protocols for Best Practice*, 3rd ed. New York, Springer Publishing.

Murphy, J., Oliver, T.M. & Cox, S. (2010) Talking Mats and Involvement in Decision Making for People with Dementia and Family Carers: Full Report. Joseph Rowntree Foundation. www.jrf.org.uk Downloaded from: http://www.jrf.org.uk/sites/files/jrf/Talking-Mats-and-decision-making-full.pdf

Office of the Public Guardian 606 (2007) Making Decisions. The Independent Mental Capacity Advocate (IMCA) Service (10.07) 2nd ed. Crown copyright. Viewed online at: https://www.gov.uk/government/uploads/system/uploads/attachment_data/file/365629/making-decisions-opg606-1207.pdf

Royal College of Speech and Language Therapy (RCSLT) (2014) SLT Provision for People with Dementia: RCSLT Position Paper. http://www.rcslt.org/members/publications/publications2/dementia_position_paper2014

Royal College of Speech and Language Therapy (RCSLT) (2014) Submission from the Royal College of Speech and Language Therapists to the Department of Health, Social Services and Public Safety and the Department of Justice's Consultation on proposals for the Draft Mental Capacity Bill, Northern Ireland. http://www.rcslt.org/governments/docs/draft_mentalcapacity_bill

Social Care Institute for Excellence. Commissioning and monitoring of Independent Mental Capacity Advocate (IMCA) services. (Viewed September 2015.) http://www.scie.org.uk/publications/guides/guide31/issues/services.asp

Social Care Institute for Excellence. IMCA Providers List (updated 2014). (Viewed September 2015). http://www.scie.org.uk/publications/imca/files/imca_providers.pdf

Talking Mats information and resources: http://www.talkingmats.com/

4 Consent, finances, discharge and other decision-making: What does the research literature say?

Anna Volkmer and Hannah Luff

Introduction

There are many different types of decisions that we make in everyday life. Some of these decisions may require more cognitive skills to manage than others. Reading and interpreting a bank statement is more difficult than counting change from a five-pound note in the newsagents. Importantly, some of these decisions may carry more risk than others. For example, deciding whether to wear a green or a blue jumper carries little risk, whilst deciding whether to give out your bank details to someone who has called up about a charitable donation may carry more significant risks.

This chapter discusses some of the more common areas that may arise in a healthcare setting with people with acquired neurological conditions, including: making medical decisions and giving consent; deciding on living situations; making financial decisions; and some other issues. We summarise the research in these areas relating to how capacity may be compromised across differing neurological conditions including dementia, aphasia and brain injury, as well as some other relevant areas. Specific examples relating to communication and dysphagia will also be included in this chapter.

Assessing capacity to consent to medical treatment

Assessing an individual's ability to consent to medical treatment is considered particularly important because of the significant risks to an individual's health and wellbeing. If the wrong decision is made, in the worst scenario this may result in unintended severe illness or death. Speech and language therapists (SLTs) can have a significant impact on this process. Maximizing an individual's comprehension can aid them in weighing up their decision appropriately, and enabling them to express their opinion will support a more mutually positive outcome. This in turn can result in a better quality of life, reduced care needs, and reduced length of admission.

Moye et al. (2007) describe consent capacity as "a patient's cognitive and emotional capacity to select among treatment alternatives or to refuse treatment" (p. 5). These authors suggest that informed consent is more distinctive than other types of capacity decisions as it arises in medical rather than legal settings and generally involves health professionals rather than lawyers. Perhaps health professionals are therefore somewhat more familiar and comfortable with this type of assessment. In reality, we are constantly assessing consent of patients to participate in therapy sessions, although these types of situations do not need the rigorous documentation that an assessment of decision-making related to a more intrusive procedure or risky operation does.

Consent is not solely an issue as regards medical procedures. Decisions about whether to go out or participate in a rehabilitative activity or whether to accept extra home or respite care are all aspects of life to which the person with dementia may or may not wish to consent (Cameron and Murphy, 2006). The NICE dementia guidelines (updated, 2011) advocate for an ongoing process of checking consent, stating that:

> "Health and social care professionals should always seek valid consent from people with dementia. This should entail informing the person of options, and checking that he or she understands, that there is no coercion and that he or she continues to consent over time. If the person lacks the capacity to make a decision, the provisions of the Mental Capacity Act 2005 must be followed." (p. 8)

This principle applies to all people with acquired neurological impairments; in fact, it applies to all people being treated at any time. Case study 1 presents some reasonably common issues around consent and capacity that can affect many patients who may be admitted to hospital.

Case Study 1

Ms Z is a woman in her 40s, who sustained a brain injury 5 years ago. She is admitted for assessment and rehabilitation. On admission to the assessment and rehabilitation unit, her decision-making ability to consent to the admission is assessed. It is felt by the treating team that she has capacity to consent to the admission. Discussion during this assessment focused on the potential gains she will make in rehabilitation and the consequent plan for her to be discharged to the optimum and most independent living situation. During the course of her admission the treating team on the ward develop a better understanding of her quite significant cognitive difficulties and feel that she will require ongoing support in a residential facility. Based on this, the team reassess her consent capacity to remain on the ward. It is now felt that she lacks capacity to make these decisions given her lack of insight into her brain injury, her care needs, her lack of recall of any information related to this and her continued preference to go to an independent living situation on finishing her time on the ward. It was consequently agreed in a best interest meetings on the ward, with her mother present, that it is in Ms Z's best interest to remain on the ward.

As previously mentioned, the MCA (2005) emphasises four core abilities required to make a consensual decision. These are:

- The ability to express a decision or choice.
- The ability to understand information related to the decision, by attending to what is said and encoding this information.
- The ability to appreciate or weigh up the information and risks related to this decision, requiring insight, foresight and judgement.
- The ability to reason and compare different alternatives through analysing and comparing information.

This seemingly straightforward process can be fraught with minefields. It can be particularly difficult to ensure people understand the impact of their decision yet avoid the use of any coercion; for example, when explaining the relevant issues related to a surgery that might in your opinion as a health professional significantly improve their quality of life, or when asking someone to participate in a piece of valuable research (Cameron et al., 2006).

The other, perhaps more clinically relevant tension, is the obligation to respect unconventional choices but protect people from harm. Enhancing the individual's ability to make a fully informed, wise (or unwise) decision is vital through the use of strategies such as: speaking slowly; not raising your voice; facing the person; giving them time; using communication aids; inviting in familiar people to support the process; repeating the discussion and allowing decisions to be considered in the person's own time. Even postponing the decision in order to treat other issues that may be confounding a person's capacity can be time efficient in the long term. Using questions that ask the individual to paraphrase a statement, summarise a discussion, explain the pro's and con's of a procedure or to reflect on the consequences of a decision are some examples of appropriate questions that might be used in this type of conversation (Lo, 1990). Lo (1990) highlights that good listening and interview skills, as well as negotiation, are essential to capacity assessments, and although seemingly time intensive, can reduce the need for more time if patients refuse treatments. Murphy et al. (2007) also found that at each session of treatment, consent will need to be revisited as many participants (with cognitive impairments) had forgotten previous discussions. This highlights the need for clinicians to revisit consent to participate in therapy sessions at each new session.

A person's capacity to make medical decisions is unique in some ways when compared to other types of capacity, in that it may not be challenged unless a patient refuses treatment that the team feels may be beneficial to them (Lo, 1990; Bellhouse et al., 2001). This means that frequently people may be mistakenly considered to have decision-making capacity simply because they 'do' or 'say' the 'right' things. One of the concerns here is that they have been inadequately assessed until the time they refuse to comply, and treatment thus may not have been delivered in the person's best interest in the past. The other dilemma is that, if the individual lacks capacity to make a decision and is refusing treatment, it can be very difficult to continue giving treatment if, for example, they are physically resisting a treatment or refusing to participate in a therapy session. This is where a decision made in that individual's best interests may still need to incorporate their wishes or that of their families, and to find evidence of what is consistent with their beliefs. For example, if someone has previously frequently declined treatments, it may not be out of character for them to refuse this treatment and may therefore be considered in their best interests. So some treatments will require both consent and capacity. The decision in this case rests with the treating doctor or other health professional. This is perhaps a familiar concept to SLTs, for example when patients refuse dysphagia management recommendations such as thickened drinks. Even if they do not have capacity to understand the risks surrounding this decision it is difficult to enforce the recommendations without the patient's consent as they can often simply refuse to drink. So, in these cases it is not uncommon that patients will continue having thin fluids following discussion with the medical team, even though there may be an associated risk (see Case study 2).

Importantly, Bellhouse et al. (2001) remind us that capacitous consent to treatment must also be informed. Therefore, the individual assessing the patient's capacity requires full knowledge of the procedure, including the benefit and risks. This means the person doing the capacity assessment must be the individual who is responsible for the treatment or procedure itself. So although SLTs may be involved in assessing an individual's skills to consent to a medical procedure or intervention it is most likely that we will be acting in a role that supports the person with communication difficulties to be able to make a decision in these cases, for example by advising team members and colleagues about the best way to present information to a person that will allow them to make an informed decision. This is an important difference compared to other types of capacity assessments. Table 4.2 provides a list of example questions for assessing decision-making abilities related to consent.

Case Study 2

Mrs H was a 98-year-old lady who lived at home with her daughter, who was also her main carer. Mrs H was deaf and partially sighted, had severe arthritis and was unable to mobilise easily. She used a four-wheel frame with supervision around her home and a wheelchair outside of the home. She had moderate vascular dementia, and had recently had a stroke that left her with swallowing difficulties. In hospital, she had been advised to take thickener in all her drinks, which she had done, but on going home she had started to refuse these. On assessment, she continued to present with difficulties tolerating thin fluids. The SLT provided an explanation of the swallow function, using a simple diagram to highlight what can happen when fluids get into the lungs and emphasised the risk of chest infections, as well as the pro's and con's of thickening fluids.

Mrs H reported that she understood this risk, but that she felt she enjoyed her cups of tea too much to continue using thickener. She stated that she had not had any chest infections to date, and that if she did that this would be acceptable to her as she was getting older. However, she acknowledged that she might reconsider her decision if she did get a chest infection in the future.

Mrs H's daughter confirmed that Mrs H had not had a chest infection to date and stated that these statements were consistent with her previous decision to stop taking thickener following her first stroke around 10 years ago, which was before she had shown any signs of cognitive deterioration or been diagnosed with dementia. The therapist liaised with Mrs H's GP, who attended a home visit with the therapist. Mrs H was unable to recall meeting the SLT before, but was able to recall the risks of fluids going down the wrong way when presented with the diagram and asked open questions, and provided the same rationale as at the previous visit. Both clinicians felt that the patient was making an informed decision consistent with her beliefs. The SLT continued to monitor Mrs H on one further visit and a follow-up telephone call. Consequently, Mrs H's daughter was given the SLT's contact details and advised to contact her should Mrs H experience any further difficulties or should she have any more concerns. Mrs H was readmitted to hospital one year later with another stroke, having not had any chest infections over that period.

What does the research say about consent and medical decision-making capacity in dementia?

There are a small number of articles in which researchers have attempted to decipher which aspects of capacity are affected in people with dementia. This has focused very much on consent capacity and on the differences between different stages of dementia. There is generally agreement amongst researchers and clinicians that these skills decline as the disease progresses (Moye et al., 2007) and that people with dementia may have some capacity in the mild stage but that this should be individually assessed. The other point which is debated in the dementia literature, is the method of assessing consent capacity. There is general agreement that formal assessment tools are not necessarily better than structured interviews. The following provides a summary of these studies.

The research tells us that the consent capacity of individuals with dementia compared to individuals without dementia is severely reduced. This is due to difficulties in the areas of understanding, but also reasoning and appreciation (Marson et al., 1995, cited in Moye et al., 2007). The same authors cite research by Marson et al. (1999) who found that people with mild Alzheimer's disease had difficulties answering questions, and frequently became confused and were unable to consider the theoretical examples given in consent capacity assessments. Moye et al. (2004) conducted a study to examine how adults with mild and moderate dementia compare to healthy control group adults on decision-making around consent capacity. The participants presented with a mixture of different dementia types. The researchers used three different formal tools with the participants that were designed to assess capacity to make medical decisions. This included the MacArthur Competence Assessment Tool for Treatment, the Hopemont Capacity Assessment Interview and the Capacity to Consent Instrument. These tools used specific questions to elicit the patients understanding of the hypothesised treatment, asked them about why they were having the treatment, why they were making the choice to have the treatment and finally rated whether they clearly expressed a decision or not. The study showed that all patients with dementia performed less well than people without dementia on measures of understanding, although patients with mild dementia generally performed within the range of normal. It also revealed that the different measures assessed appreciation very differently, resulting in most people with dementia passing this on one test and on another test many of the control group failing. Similarly, the different measures were inconsistent in their rating of reasoning across both the control and dementia groups. Finally, the study found that all participants with mild and moderate dementia were able to express a decision or choice on all measures. Moye et al. (2004) concluded that assessment tools should be interpreted with a focus on individual situations and be facilitated by use of strategies to compensate for impairments. They highlighted that clinical situations are often not structured strictly as formal evaluations so the use of notes, diagrams and references is common; similarly, the use of communication aids to facilitate comprehension for aphasic people will be common.

Perhaps one of the most concerning findings from the literature is that it is not only formal assessments that demonstrate reduced reliability across tools, but also that clinicians completing informal structured interviews to assess consent capacity demonstrate little agreement on whether or not patients had capacity (Marson et al., 1995, cited in Moye et al., 2007). Moye et al. (2007) attribute this to the fact that measurement strategies developed for one patient may work less well with other patients. They summarise a number of studies that examine the association between capacity measures and cognitive measures for different conditions. They found that different factors predicted difficulties on different tasks; for example, patients with Alzheimer's dementia who had difficulties with conceptualisation, verbal fluency and naming demonstrated difficulties in understanding, appreciating and reasoning related to a medical decision. On the other hand, patients with Parkinson's dementia who had executive difficulties and memory impairments demonstrated most difficulty in understanding and reasoning related to a decision. However, the authors emphasise that, with training, clinicians can demonstrate increased reliability. Moye et al. (2007) also reflect on the different skills that different clinicians bring to capacity assessments and urge that these different approaches need to be explored.

What does the research say about consent and medical decision-making in aphasia?

Clinical "researchers have a vested interest in gaining consent from their subjects, but do they protect their interests?" ask Kagan and Kimelman (1995, p. 66). They suggest that SLTs have not made the rights of aphasic patients a priority. And although the literature in this area is increasing, this remains a fairly 'young' issue in the aphasia literature. Indeed Morris et al. (2012) estimate that no research was done in the area of stroke and decision-making capacity until 2005. This means that what articles there are in the literature generally focus on capturing case examples and clinical opinions.

It will not be surprising to SLTs that there may be particular challenges in balancing respect for autonomy of an aphasic person with the need to have a comprehensive discussion of the risks and benefits of a medical intervention in order to establish consent capacity (Stein & Wagner, 2006). Decision-making capacity may well be preserved in people with aphasia, yet the patients' ability to fully participate in a 'traditional' verbal dialogue regarding a proposed medical intervention may be impaired. (Kagan & Kimelman, 1995; Stein & Wagner, 2006). Frequently people with aphasia may have treatment-related decisions made for them or are excluded from research studies altogether (Townend et al., 2007, Jayes & Palmer, 2014). Excluding people with aphasia from research studies is not only unethical but may mean people with aphasia do not receive the same standards of health care. It is therefore also not surprising that much research examining the development of formal assessments of capacity to consent have excluded people with aphasia (Aldous et al., 2014).

Excluding individuals with aphasia from decision-making should not be the routine method of managing these situations for people with aphasia, many of whom are able to make decisions given the opportunity and the right environment. Indeed, Kagan and Kimelman (1995) asked people with aphasia if others should make decisions for them, and more than 50% of those people said "No". Of the respondents, 76% agreed that in order to make decisions standard consent forms should be altered to suit their needs.

Many researchers have highlighted the importance of informed consent forms being written in language that is understandable to the participant (Metz & Folkins, 1985; Sachs & Cassell, 1990; Kagan & Kimelman, 1995). They also highlight the value of testing comprehension and not assuming it because someone has 'made all the correct noises'. Indeed, people with aphasia may have intact social and pragmatic skills which enable them to nod at all the correct times, masking their incapacity. Testing this type of comprehension using yes or no verification questions is advocated by many aphasiologists (Kagan & Kimelman, 1995).

Jayes and Palmer (2014) recently conducted a survey to assess what happens in real research practice for people with language impairments. The vast majority of researchers seeking consent report using conversation to identify communication difficulties (91%), with only a few reporting that they use specific screening tools (12%). Only 4% suggested that they would seek SLT support. About a third of respondents reported they did not use accessible information and consent forms as they are not available, and 20% report not supporting their conversations with any adaptations such as gestures or drawing as they have not had any training in this area. Of those surveyed, 65% had received training from an SLT and identified learning and practising the use of strategies to support people with aphasia in their communication as most useful. Overall, seeking consent from this patient group was considered difficult and time consuming.

Aldous et al. (2014) recently conducted a survey to explore the common practices of SLTs involved in the assessment of decision-making capacity for clients with aphasia in clinical situations. They found that, of those SLTs who responded to their survey, 86% had been involved in the assessment of decision-making for a patient with aphasia and the majority of those were based in acute inpatient and inpatient rehabilitation settings. This may perhaps be because this is the setting where the majority of treatment consent decisions take place. Indeed, more respondents indicated they were frequently involved in assessing decision-making related to health and medical decisions compared to other types of decisions. Aldous et al. (2014) found that SLTs use a wide variety of assessment methods and tools, including informal and formal testing, and discussions with the treating team and the family around the individual. Clinicians reported focusing on verbal comprehension and expression as well as reading and writing, and strategies to support conversation. Most reported not using formal assessment tools, but those that did used the Western Aphasia Battery, the Mt Wilga Higher Level Language Test, the Cognitive Linguistic Quick Test and a selection of other commonly-used language assessments. Hence, Aldous et al. (2014) recommend there is not a 'one size fits all' approach to formal assessments of decision-making capacity for people with aphasia, but there would be much value in the formulation of guidelines and principles for capacity evaluation to support SLTs on developing competencies which may in turn improve their confidence in this area of clinical practice. Furthermore, Jayes and Palmer (2014) emphasise the need for training of other staff members in communication strategies as a way of reducing the barriers for people with aphasia to be able to engage in consent processes.

There have been some attempts to design tools to support the assessment of people with aphasia, namely the consent support tool (CST) developed by Jayes and Palmer (2013). The tool involves an informal screening test of an individual's comprehension of spoken and written language, through a series of tasks including carrying out commands, identifying objects and reading a passage. Performance is then linked to four specific profiles that provide guidance on how to present information, for example, "if s/he is able to read three key words (words that convey salient information) in a sentence, information should be formatted using the aphasia-friendly recommendations proposed by Connect (2007)" (Jayes & Palmer, 2013, p. 2). Jayes and Palmer found that in their small sample of 13 adults with aphasia their tool accurately predicted the appropriate level of communication required in 11 of their participants. The types of strategies that may be suggested are discussed further in the next chapter.

What does the research say about consent and medical decision-making capacity in brain injury?

There are some researchers who have attempted to identify the cognitive impairments most associated with issues of consent capacity for people who have had a brain injury. Dreer et al. (2008) examined cognitive predictors of medical decision-making capacity in participants with a brain injury at time of acute injury (baseline) and at a six-month follow-up using a consent capacity instrument (Capacity to Consent to Treatment Instrument: CCTI) and neuropsychological test measures. Although they found multiple cognitive skills associated with impaired medical decision-making capacity, impairments of short-term verbal memory were strongly associated with impairments in consent capacity at the time of acute injury. As patients experience cognitive and functional recovery post-hospitalisation, executive functioning and working memory abilities were associated with improved capacity at six-month follow-up. This emphasises the increased likelihood of patients requiring support whilst admitted to acute hospital settings immediately after a injury. Marson et al. (2005) also found that patients with brain injury showed initial impairment and subsequent partial recovery of medical decision making capacity over a six-month period. Complex consent abilities of appreciation, reasoning, and understanding were significantly impaired in hospitalised acute brain injury patients. At 6 months post-injury, the same individuals showed substantial recovery of reasoning and partial recovery of appreciation and understanding consent abilities. The researchers here also emphasise the importance of re-assessing consent capacity in the rehabilitation setting for people with brain injuries. This idea of re-assessment in the rehabilitation setting is likely also relevant to the majority of our aphasic patients.

Other researchers have examined different severities of brain injury and the associations with how these individuals perform on the four domains of an assessment of medical decision-making capacity. Triebel et al. (2012) investigated medical decision-making capacity in patients with acute brain injury across a range of injury severity one month after injury. They found that people with a mild brain injury performed similarly to controls on all domains, whilst some people with more complex, but still mild brain injuries demonstrated more difficulties in understanding. People with moderate or severe brain injuries were impaired in all domains, and more impaired than complex mild brain injuries in comprehension. This highlights that some people with mild brain injuries may particularly benefit from support from an SLT, or a professional who has been appropriately trained to modify the information and how it is presented to maximise the opportunities for these people to understand the information given.

Recognising the needs of someone with a brain injury can be quite complex.

Brain injury is often described as a 'hidden disability'. Indeed, an individual can 'mask' their difficulties in a one-off assessment of decision-making capacity, and may require a more dynamic, informed process. In clinical practice, it is the risks that can arise as a result of not recognising these cognitive issues which are perhaps most concerning. A report by the Acquired Brain Injury and Mental Capacity Act Interest Group House of Lords Select Committee Post-Legislative Scrutiny Report into the Mental Capacity Act in 2014 stated:

> "…consequences of acquired brain injury are often invisible and can be subtle but devastating for the sufferer and their family and community. People are often left fatigued, with slowed speed of processing, difficulties with attention (divided, sustained, selective etc.), with memory, planning, organising, initiating activity, problem solving, with rigidity of thinking, disinhibited behaviour, predicting and understanding the consequences of one's actions, impulsivity and aggression. The sufferer rarely has complete insight into their condition." (p. 4)

The report emphasises that unskilled professionals often do not understand issues around lack of insight, i.e. the difference between the person saying what he believes he can do and what he can actually do. Thus they recommend that any assessments of decision-making capacity for people with brain injury should be conducted by or with a professional with expertise in the area of brain injury (such as an SLT) or alongside a family member with an understanding of this person's limitations. These assessments often require more than one discrete meeting; instead, a dynamic process of assessment of the individual's areas of cognitive strength and difficulties. The report flags a real risk of local authorities, social workers and advocates (specifically Independent Mental Capacity Advocates) misjudging these cognitive limitations for the right to make a poor decision. They describe cases of this resulting in neglect and risk in the provision of care and support to vulnerable adults.

What does the research say about consent and decision-making in adults with learning difficulties (ALD)?

ALD encompasses a wide range of different abilities and communication styles and methods. For people with milder learning difficulties, there is evidence that they are able to consent and be involved in decision-making across many domains. Inglis and Cook (2011) looked at engaging people with ALD in research and, as a result, provided 10 'top tips' to assist other researchers in engaging this client group. They noted that research is often about adults with a learning difficulty rather than research done in collaboration with adults with a learning difficulty. Key points that they raised, which have direct relevance to other aspects of decision-making capacity were (p. 101–102):

- There should be a presumption of capacity

- One type of information event is unlikely to be enough – that is, information may need to be presented in different ways over time

- Not everyone knows what questions to ask before consenting

- Engaging the participants and their significant others may be helpful

- Not everyone may understand the implications of saying "no".

Skinner et al. (2010) published an article on assessing the treatment consent capacity of adults with learning difficulties. The authors were part of a multidisciplinary team (Capacity Assessment Team) who set up a service model for assessing the consent capacity of adults with learning difficulties referred to ophthalmology for intervention. They describe setting up a screening system, which considered the individual's communication skills, their mental health status and understanding of the decision using an initial accessible leaflet. They also report using a full assessment, which included open questions, contextual discussions of recent hospital admissions, semi-structured interviewing techniques and vignettes once patients had passed the initial screening phase. If the patient failed the initial screening phase the medical team were advised of this, and recommendations made to proceed in the patient's best interests. In this case, the team would offer to support this best interest decision. If the patient demonstrated capacity they would be supported to attend their medical appointment, where the consent would be confirmed by the medical team using the appropriately developed supports (e.g. picture cards).

Where individuals have profound and complex needs, there can be a clear lack of capacity. While no other adult is able to consent for medical treatment on another's behalf, unless there is a lasting power of attorney for health and welfare decisions, families of people with severe learning difficulties have often strongly advocated for their relative over many years. These experiences may not have been positive, with one relative stating to Goldbart and Barton (2010) in their study for Mencap:

> "How can you trust them [medical professionals] when they're trying to write her off all the time?" (p. 21)

When best interests decisions are being made, it is therefore vital to listen to family and to be aware of their previous experiences with health and social care services. A single case study by Kiani et al. (2014) used reflective practice and an analysis of the literature to look at barriers to cancer care for people with ALD. They analysed barriers relating to the service user, the service itself and healthcare professionals and carers. The importance of using a wide range of communication tools with people with ALD was highlighted and this is further explored by Goldbart and Caton (2010).

For a detailed case analysis of complex decision-making that resonates for the adult population, although it concerns a child with severe physical and learning difficulties, Radio 4's "Inside the Ethics Committee" has a thought-provoking discussion of a real-life case, with perspectives gathered from the mother and the team working with the child. It highlights the experiences that many carers of people with ALD may have faced in their interactions with health care professionals and the communication barriers that need to be overcome.

What does the research say about decision-making in other conditions

Many studies looking at decisions in Motor Neurone Disease (MND) focus more on having a voice and the timing of discussions around non-oral feeding and end-of-life support rather than on whether people with MND have capacity to make these decisions. There have been some efforts to deal with this issue more recently in the MND literature. Hogden et al. (2012) interviewed 37 health professionals working with people with MND, and 75% of respondents reported that cognitive and behavioural changes impacted on patients' health care decision-making. They found that "the effects of subtle cognitive and behavioural change on decision-making were not easily specified" (p. 694). Participants stated that patients frequently retained the capacity to make decisions. Nevertheless, "the quality and timing of their decisions appeared compromised by a lack of motivation, and limited insight into their condition and the needs of their families" (p.694). Many patients were described as being 'difficult' and having rigid personalities, particularly by clinicians working in the palliative phase of care. Because cognitive and behavioural change was not routinely assessed in the clinics, identification of patients at risk of impaired decision-making skills was neither systematic nor standardised. Health professionals explained that more specific and detailed knowledge of these changes could improve their approach with the patient and carer and allow them to broach advanced care planning at the most appropriate points (Hogden et al., 2012). This issue of advanced care planning and capacity is further discussed in Chapter 7.

Although the impact of patients' cognitive and behavioral deterioration on decision-making in people with MND remains undefined, Hogden et al. (2013) have done work with carers who also considered that the patient's lack of insight placed significant strains on decision-making. This mirrors some of the literature on brain injury, which emphasises the importance of insight to decision-making capacity.

Kleeberg et al. (2004) have examined the impact of decision-making in 20 people with Multiple Sclerosis (MS). They assessed their decision-making using the Iowa Gambling Task. The authors initially hypothesised that intrahemispheric functional disconnection of the prefrontal cortex from other brain regions then could be expected to occur in MS and thus affect decision-making. On analysing the results, they found that people with MS who struggled with decision-making also demonstrated delayed learning. Other researchers have attributed the same decision-making difficulties to mood disorders in MS (Simioni et al., 2009). More recently Muhlert et al. (2015) found that gauging risk and adapting accordingly (risk adjustment), and slow deliberation rather than impulsivity, were the primary features of impaired decision-making in MS. They found no evidence for increased impulsivity in MS. Muhlert et al. (2015) recommend that, since decision-making impairment was seen in people with MS who did not show other cognitive deficits, specific assessments are required to detect issues in the context of real-life decision-making.

Decision-making capacity to manage finances

Assessing an individual's decision-making capacity to manage their own finances is considered particularly important due to the significant risks to an individual's wellbeing. If the patient makes the wrong decisions they may be left vulnerable to unpaid bills, debt build-up and bankruptcy, as well as increased vulnerability to scams. SLTs can have a significant role in this process, both as assessors and facilitators. The SLT may also be involved in supporting the individual to understand the rationale for the assessment, and enabling them to express preferences about who they would like to support them in managing their finances in the future should they be found to lack capacity in this area.

The capacity to manage financial affairs is considered a fundamental instrumental activity of daily living "critical to independent functioning of adults in our society" (Marson et al., 2000). Marson et al. also emphasise that it is "possibly the best single litmus for capacity to live independently". Legally speaking, financial capacity may be applied only to the skills required to manage ones own finances and estate (Marson et al., 2012).

Moye et al. (2007) describe financial capacity as "a broad range of conceptual, pragmatic and judgment abilities". This includes skills ranging from counting and checking coins and cash, using a cash point and writing cheques, as well as checking and managing bank statements and bills, writing a will and deciding on financial investments. It is important to remember that a person's level of finance management skill will vary widely in cognitively-intact individuals based on many factors including education, occupation and socio-economic status (Marson et al., 2012).

Dreer et al. (2012) highlight that impairment in mental and written arithmetic, reduced semantic financial knowledge, poor self-awareness, insight, impulsivity, disinhibition and short-term memory difficulties can all negatively influence financial decision-making. Financial capacity requires three particular types of knowledge and skills. First, having declarative knowledge which is the ability to describe information related to financial activities such as knowing how much money is paid into one's account every month from one's wage or benefits. The second skill is the procedural knowledge (or performance aspect) required to carry out financially-related tasks such as writing a cheque. Third, there is judgement; the skill of making appropriate decisions to protects one's financial interests (Marson et al., 2000).

This range of skills can be considered a spectrum, where one person may be able to manage small amounts of monies, e.g. once given some cash they may be able to go to the shops and purchase a small amount of items, also checking their change appropriately. This person may only need support for bigger financial tasks such as managing their accounts and paying bills. In comparison, a different person may require more assistance to manage all aspects of their monies. If an individual does need support, it is important to engage them in conversation to identity whom they would prefer to provide them with the required support. This is a key area of the financial capacity assessment as it can not only reveal their level of insight, but also provide them with the opportunity for choice and support. This is where it is key to ensure a patient with communication impairment is able to express a preference if possible, as patients are more likely to consent and comply with recommendations if they have been able to voice a choice of some kind.

The MCA (2005) does not require the use of formal instrumental assessments, although there are instruments that have been developed with this in mind. The Financial Capacity Instrument (FCI) is a standardised measure of performance on financial tasks with direct relevance to the demands of everyday money management. It examines performance across six domains: monetary skills, conceptual knowledge, cash transactions, cheque book management, bank statement management and financial judgement. People with mild Alzheimer's have been found to perform as well as age-matched controls on simpler tasks but less well on more complex tasks on this test. The Measure of Awareness of Financial Skills (MAFS) is a similar test but also addresses patient insight and carer concerns. Some authors suggest that this type of test can provide relevant information, above that given by standard cognitive assessments (Moberg & Pick, 2008). It could be perceived that these types of areas may be assessed in functionally relevant occupational therapy or speech and language therapy tests. Indeed, the Communication Activities of Daily Living assessment tool for aphasia includes tasks related to basic money and bill handling, as does the Functional Reading Test. Yet, semi-structured interviews are still likely to form part of the assessment process and Table 6.2 provides a list of example questions for assessing decision-making abilities related to finances.

What does the research say about financial decision-making capacity in dementia?

It is worth mentioning the literature on financial capacity in adults with dementia, even though it is sparse and only recently emerging. There is evidence from assessments of adults with mild Alzheimer's dementia that they will have difficulties in both simple and more complex financial tasks and, perhaps more concerningly, a lack of insight to this difficulty (Moye et al., 2007). There is also evidence that people with mild cognitive impairment (MCI) will start to demonstrate difficulties in these areas compared to healthy adults of the same age (Griffith et al., 2003). This is important as it is generally assumed that people with MCI are able to manage much more independently than people with dementia, yet evidence shows they are already becoming vulnerable in this area of daily life.

What does the research say about financial decision-making capacity in aphasia?

There is even less literature available on how people with aphasia manage financial decision-making. However, there is general agreement in the non-speech and language therapy literature that people with aphasia perform poorly on formal assessment tools of financial capacity, particularly if there an impairment of language comprehension involved (Heilbronner, 2011). This will not be a surprise to any SLT, and only highlights that people with aphasia are generally excluded from the research literature on decision-making capacity.

Interestingly, SLTs who responded to Aldous et al's (2014) survey on current clinical practices in the assessment of decision-making capacity reported they were least likely to be involved in assessments of financial decision-making when compared to other types of decisions. This is perhaps a consequence of the differing cognitive processes involved in finances. Stroke psychologists report that, of the capacity referrals that they are asked to complete, financial decision-making accounts for 14%, the second most common issue after placement (Morris et al., 2012). It may be the psychologist or occupational therapist who has been examining an individual's arithmetic or money handling, or a social worker who is fully informed of the individual's current financial issues and income who conducts this capacity assessment. Consequently, the presence of another health professional is perhaps overwhelming. This reinforces the need for SLTs to equip and train their colleagues in the multidisciplinary team with the skills they require to manage this person's communication.

It is interesting to compare these reports from the stroke and aphasia literature to that from the progressive aphasia literature. Kindell et al's (2015) study collected consensus opinions from expert practitioners working with progressive aphasia, specifically semantic dementia. These clinicians did report being involved in assessments of decision-making capacity for finances, as well as consent, care, driving, and power of attorney related decisions. They highlight the SLT's role as either directly doing the capacity assessment or "supporting the person's participation through simplifying information, written prompts, and utilizing preserved areas of understanding to explain issues". It is hypothesised that this difference between the involvement of SLTs in assessments of financially-related decision-making in progressive versus non-progressive aphasias is related to the multidisciplinary team involved more than the decision itself.

What does the research say about financial decision-making capacity in brain injury?

There is currently a little more research addressing assessment of capacity to manage personal finances in the brain injury literature. Some of this research focuses on the patterns of cognitive impairments that tally up with impairments of decision-making capacity in this area.

Hoskin et al. (2005) investigated whether neuropsychological assessment could assist in determining capacity to manage personal finances in people who have had a brain injury. They compared a group of people with brain injury who were currently independently managing their personal finances with a group of people with brain injury who had been deemed to lack decision-making capacity and were being supported in these tasks, for example by an assigned deputy. The second group performed significantly worse than the first group on measures of executive and attentional skills (impulse control, planning, flexibility of thinking and working memory). However, there were no significant differences between groups on measures of memory. McHugh and Wood (2008) confirmed impulsivity as a contributor to impairments of financial decision-making in people with brain injuries. Martin et al. (2012) compared healthy controls to people with moderate-to-severe brain injuries immediately post injury and again six months later. In particular, arithmetic, working memory, and immediate verbal memory were impaired in people who lacked financial capacity immediately post injury, whilst at 6 months mental arithmetic and working memory skills remained impaired in those who still lacked capacity.

In the report by the Acquired Brain Injury and Mental Capacity Act Interest Group for the House of Lords Select Committee Post-Legislative Scrutiny Report into the Mental Capacity Act (2014) it is flagged that "in practice, in a structured and guided conversation led by a well-intentioned and intelligent other, such as a social worker, brain injured people with intellectual awareness and reasonably intact IQ can frequently demonstrate good understanding in relation to decisions relating to matters of finance... in doing so, the test for the assessment of capacity, according to the Mental Capacity Act and guidance, would appear to be met" (p. 24). They caution that these types of conversations can be misleading with people who have had a brain injury. The authors emphasise that, when it comes to real-life events, people with brain injuries frequently lack financial decision-making capacity. In other words, though someone with a brain injury may say they would do one thing (demonstrating capacity), they consequently do another thing. The report also highlights a real reluctance from other services to challenge this shallow appearance of capacity for fear of the related social costs, for example in assigning financial deputies.

That said, a large number of people with brain injuries are likely to be living with their loved ones, who would be involved in joint decision-making. Some researchers are focusing on these relationships, to understand the effective components of this decision making relationship (Knox et al., 2015). This will provide useful 'real' insights that will contribute to the future support of families in the clinical setting, as illustrated by Case study 3.

Case Study 3

Mr X lived at home with his wife prior to his admission to the assessment ward with suspected fronto-temporal dementia on the background of a brain injury. Mr X had sustained a brain injury after falling down the stairs of his home three years ago. He was in his mid 50s and lived at home with his wife, and his three teenage children. Mrs X reported that over the last 2 months Mr X had become increasingly aggressive and suspicious. He had threatened her and on one occasion he had also threatened their son. She also reported that he appeared to forget things more often, and had recently got lost on a few occasions on the way home from the shops he goes to every week. She reported that prior to Mr X's brain injury he had managed all their finances, but that since his injury she had taken over this responsibility as his deputy. Recently, he had hidden a number of bills and statements before she had been able to get to the post, and had become very frustrated and agitated when she refused to allow him to apply for credit cards. Mrs X stated that this was an area which was causing increasing concern (among other concerns) and although she wished him to return home she felt he couldn't return to managing the finances but was unsure how to communicate this to him. During his admission the occupational therapist (OT), psychologist and SLT reviewed Mr X's ability to manage his finances. This involved:

• Liaising with Mrs X about the family banking (including bank where account held, benefit details, etc), managing small change at the shops and discussing how Mr X had managed these prior to his injury, e.g. was he frugal, or often in debt?

- Asking Mr X about his knowledge of the family assets and income, etc.
- Asking him to participate in functional assessment with the OT using small monies at the shops.
- Assessment of his ability to read a bill and identify important information relevant to payment and checking information was accurate.
- Asking Mr X to explain his rationale for applying for two credit cards and why he supposed his wife was unhappy about this.
- Discussing the benefits and disadvantages to having a credit card.
- Asking him how he would manage if he ran into difficulties using vignette examples of what could go wrong.

Assessment indicated that Mr X continued to lack capacity to manage his and the family's finances, although he was able to manage small amounts of money when going to the shops to buy a few items. He was unable to attend to the task and demonstrated reduced attention in reading a bill to check information as accurate. Mr X was also unable to weigh up the risks around applying for a credit card, or plan how he would make repayments. However, the team felt it would be useful for his wife to be able to involve him in the task of managing the bills, as it had previously been part of his role. Together with Mrs X, the team devised a structured method whereby Mr X was able to sit with his wife reading out bill information, whilst she completed the banking tasks and reported on what she was doing. Mr and Mrs X reported ongoing satisfaction in this task six months after discharge.

Decision-making capacity to decide on living situation

Assessing an individual's decision-making capacity to decide on their discharge destination or ability to live independently is considered particularly important due to the significant risks to an individual's physical health. There are also risks to their social wellbeing to consider. If the patient makes the wrong decisions here it may result in them not being able to manage basic care tasks such as taking medications and feeding themselves (self-neglect). It can also have implications for managing high-risk situations, such as if there was a fire in their home. This could ultimately lead to death or serious illness. SLTs can have a significant impact on this assessment process, again as both assessors and facilitators.

Deciding on discharge destination or living situation is considered a vast area of functioning that can cover almost all aspects of daily living skills, from basic daily care such as washing, personal hygiene and dressing to cooking, buying food and keeping the home clean and habitable. There are also more complex things to consider such as ability and safety awareness in the local community, cognition and navigation around the community, as well as problem-solving skills such as the ability to call for help when needed. Moye et al. (2007) highlight that this area of need often goes unrecognised and is misunderstood, particularly when considering risks such as neglect and withdrawal from services.

This is an area where the SLT can also act as both assessor and facilitator. Indeed, assessing an individual's ability to communicate on the phone in a potential emergency situation, speak to shop assistants to get what they need, and communicate with their local care providers, such as their GP, about how they are managing may be key parts of the assessment process. As with the area of consent capacity the SLT can have an important role in supporting a patient to understand the options available to them, and make an informed decision about where they would like to live. It is also vital that the patient is afforded the option of highlighting where he or she would prefer to live. Table 6.2 provides a list of example questions for assessing decision-making abilities related to discharge.

As previously discussed in reference to consent capacity it can be difficult to enforce a decision made by someone other than the patient, if the patient does not consent to such as a specific living situation. And although there are ways of supporting this, it can be difficult to maintain this environment, and can impact significantly on an individual's wellbeing. This option must be carefully considered. The Deprivation of Liberty Safeguards (DoLS) was introduced in 2007 as part of the MCA (2005). DoLS apply to people who suffer from a "mental disorder or disability of the mind", such as dementia, who lack the capacity to give informed consent for the arrangements made for their care and/or treatment. In these cases, it may be that depriving them of their liberty is necessary and in their best interests in order to protect them from harm. The safeguards cover patients in hospitals and people in care homes.

DoLS are designed to protect the interests of a person, to ensure that they are given the care they need in the least restrictive environment, so preventing them from being deprived of their liberty.

What does the research say about living situation and decision-making capacity in aphasia?

There is little in the way of research on the area of aphasia and discharge decisions, although marginally more than that related to financial decision-making. This seems to align itself appropriately with clinical reports; indeed, in Aldous et al.'s (2014) survey of SLTs respondents reported they were sometimes involved in assessing decision-making in relation to lifestyle issues but less than when compared to medical decision-making.

The majority of people who have an aphasia resulting from a stroke will have been admitted to hospital at some point. Many of these have consequently spent some time in a rehabilitation unit. A small study of 34 stroke rehabilitation inpatients found that 35% did not have capacity to make a decision about their own discharge (Mackenzie et al., 2008). The researchers found no significant difference in any aspect of cognitive functioning between stroke patients who did or did not have decision-making capacity in relation to discharge destination. They also found that not only is performance on cognitive test scores a poor predictor of capacity to decide on discharge destination, but age and dysphasia are not good predictors either in stroke patients receiving rehabilitation.

According to Dickey et al. (2010), twice as many patients with stroke and aphasia were discharged to long-term care than those who presented with stroke alone. This raises concerns as to whether these people's decision-making is being fairly assessed. Aside from any unnecessary restriction on personal liberty that this may present, any barriers to consent and discharge have financial implications for health and social care in addition to personal cost.

A standardised capacity assessment for admission to long-term care does not exist (Carling-Rowland et al., 2014). Yet social workers are considered to be the gold standard capacity evaluators because of their training in capacity legislation, not making assumptions and viewing a patient as a whole person rather than a diagnosis (Hepworth et al., 2006, cited in Carling-Rowland, 2014). Carling-Rowland et al. (2014) describe the Communication Aid to Capacity Evaluation (CACE)'s development and validation with a group of social workers, assessing people with aphasia on decision-making with regards to long-term care. They trained the social workers to use the CACE and introduced them to supportive communication techniques. They found that the structure and support offered by the CACE helped the people with aphasia understand the purpose and content of the capacity assessment, resulting in accurate determination of their capacity. They found that the structure of the tool reduced inconsistencies across individual tests in how information was presented. The average age of the people with aphasia in this study was 62 years; the researcher emphasises that this is lower than the mean age of people living in long-term residential care, and so assessing the decision-making of an individual in relation to this change in living circumstances is all the more important both emotionally, socially and financially. The researchers note that, in this research study, it was not the person with aphasia who owned the communication barrier but rather the assessor's skills and confidence which were the stumbling block. This only serves to emphasise the important role of SLTs in training others, and conducting assessments themselves.

It is also worth referring back to the idea of domains of 'performance' capacity versus 'judgement' capacity that were highlighted in the previous section on financial capacity. Here, we explained that people might be able to perform certain tasks such as managing a weekly budget but not the finer details of their bank account. In the same way, clinicians in practice will assess a person's ability to buy the correct foods, prepare them, call the ambulance and care for themselves on a day-to-day basis in comparison to verbally explaining this. It will be very difficult to verbally explain these in a discussion with a person with aphasia, yet they may well be able to demonstrate these skills, with support for higher-level tasks such as taking medications regularly. Using functional tasks and weekend leave can form part of a multidimensional capacity assessment (Mukherjee & McDonough, 2006).

What does the research say about living situation and decision-making capacity in brain injury?

There is currently very little research addressing assessment of decision-making around the living situation in the brain injury literature. It seems that sometimes this area is entrenched within medical decision-making and care. Again, some of this research focuses on the patterns of cognitive impairments that tally up with the four domains of decision-making capacity, whilst other resources focus more on the clinical reality and the risks surrounding this type of decision-making.

Owen et al. (2015) examined the decision-making capacity skills (including discharge decisions) in a series of case studies of people with brain injuries and organic personality disorders. They highlight that awareness of deficit and "thinking about thinking" can be present without being "effectively available for use in decision-making". The authors provide advice around the type of information to collect prior to the capacity assessment itself, including gathering information on previous potentially 'unwise' decisions and collecting a collateral on personality changes since the injury. They also recommend considering whether a patient can demonstrate an awareness of their deficits:

- Is it online awareness?

- Is the person able to make *use* of his or her awareness in the context of deliberating?

- How does the person respond to his or her impulses in the context of decision-making and action?

- Does the person have the ability to resolve or disengage from impulses that may arise in a decision situation?

- To what extent is the person able to use his or her feelings, or to what extent are they influenced by their feelings when faced with a decision?

These suggestions do not form a definitive list but are worth reflecting on during the assessment process.

Mukherjee and McDonough (2006) investigated the ways health care providers address issues of decision-making capacity on a daily basis with people with brain injuries. They conducted semi-structures focus groups with a total of 33 rehabilitation clinicians from eight different occupations. All agreed that decision-making capacity was a consideration in their daily practice. Participants emphasised the need for a 'multidimensional' rather than a 'unitary' definition of decision-making capacity and the need to be aware of fluctuating capacities due to the injury. The participants also highlighted the importance not just of the person's own safety but of the health care provider and community members when considering discharge. The authors concluded that this specific type of decision-making is dependent on the unique context of each individual's home situation, their actual abilities and the risks involved.

Finally, the report by the Acquired Brain Injury and Mental Capacity Act Interest Group for the House of Lords Select Committee Post-Legislative Scrutiny Report into the Mental Capacity Act (2014) states that "Privileging notions of 'independence' may possibly be unrealistic for those with cognitive, executive or behavioural difficulties following brain injury and removes notions of reintegration (Willer et al., 1993) that, it may be argued, are more accurate descriptors of the way non-brain injured people live and fails to take account of risks from the wider community"(p. 27). This concept of community risk is similar to that described by Mukherjeee and McDonough (2006). These authors raise the issue of insight as a barrier to appropriate decision-making capacity for people with brain injury and provide clinical examples. They describe how people with brain injuries may be assessed as having decision-making capacity in discrete 'assessments', yet be unable to perform in reality due to their lack of insight and self-monitoring. This can put individuals at high risk of self-neglect, vulnerability from others and have a significant impact on both their quality of life and their wellbeing. This also ties in with the recent research by Owen et al. (2015). Structured environments such as those offered by supported accommodation will provide a platform to minimise these risks and the positive impact of these cannot be underestimated. Indeed, the report provides an example of an individual who had been severely neglectful of his own health and home, whose behaviour and wellbeing were improved in a structured environment, with staff who were able to continue to provide him with appropriate choices in his daily living, using accessible language. Mr J in case study 4 is a similar example of such a case.

Case Study 4

Mr J was a man in his late 50s who contracted HIV some years ago, He had been living alone in the community until recently but had not been taking his medications. This had led to a deterioration in his health and admission to hospital. He had continued to deteriorate in hospital, refusing medications and becoming increasingly unmanageable. Mr J was transferred from the hospital, where they were struggling to manage his increasingly aggressive behaviour and agitation. He was admitted to specialist care and sectioned as it was felt he was psychotic. He also presented with significant cognitive and communication difficulties.

During the course of his admission he started to take his medication again and as he became more well his cognition and communication improved somewhat. On imaging, however, it was felt that he presented with white matter changes consistent with HIV dementia. On making plans for his consequent discharge from the unit, a home visit was conducted. Due to the unsanitary conditions and general state of disrepair it was highlighted that his home was not safe to be lived in. The team also felt that Mr J's physical and cognitive difficulties would mean he would require 24-hour support and supervision. During the course of his admission Mr J expressed a desire to return to his home.

He had brothers who were involved in discussion around discharge and reported that he had always lived in what others considered to be unsanitary conditions. They were unable to provide the support he required, and local mental and disability services also stated they would not be able to support this either.

The SLT and psychologist conducted an initial capacity assessment, using a structured interview model, to examine his ability to make decisions related to discharge. On assessment, Mr J insisted that he wished to return home, and that he did not believe his physical or cognitive difficulties would prevent him from managing safely. He stated that he would likely discontinue taking his medications if he went home, but that this was okay, as he did not feel they were helping. Mr J refused further discussion on this topic. At a later date, the therapists returned to review this assessment. At this point, the clinicians explained the team's concern about his welfare and advised Mr J of what we were recommending, providing some written and pictoral information of recommended residential homes in the area. It was also suggested that he could return to his home to visit and collect his belongings. Mr J stated that he understood the team were concerned about his welfare and agreed that he wanted to remain well, stating that the support from the staff at the unit would likely be helpful. He consented to the referral being made and was keen to visit his home.

Although Mr J's feelings about the residential center continued to fluctuate, he remained agreeable to this plan in further similar conversations using written and pictoral supports. He was able to visit his home to collect his belongings. Upon visiting his home he expressed surprise at the state of his home but insisted that he felt he could have lived there independently and that he was not unwell, although he understood the team's recommendations were around keeping him as well as possible.

The team agreed that Mr J lacked the capacity to make this decision. At this time, it was felt his needs would be best met in specialist care and he was later discharged to one of the residential units in which he had expressed an interest. During his admission to hospital, Mr J has been detained under the Mental Health Act, but this was revised on his discharge and the team at the residential facility applied for a Deprivation of Liberty Safeguard.

Table 4.1 Example questions for capacity assessment (this is not an exhaustive list by any means and just provides some ideas).

NB: These questions have not been modified for anyone with receptive language difficulties or a cognitive communication difficulty. Chapter 4 describes in detail the tools and strategies that can be used to modify language and make assessments more accessible. This table is simply a guide to the types of things you may wish to find out/ask in some way.

It is also important to be aware the difference between performance capacity and judgement capacity which is described in the text above. This table does not provide an exhaustive list of either of these areas.

	Assessment questions (examples)
Consent capacity	Explain area of medical concern and recommended treatment. Advise patient of alternatives to recommended treatment. Provide information on risks of treatment and risks of choosing alternatives.
	Ask patient to recall/repeat/rephrase or summarise this information.
	What is your preference?
	Why do you prefer that option?
	What do you think are the pro's and con's of treatment/the alternatives to the recommended treatment?

	Appelbaum (2007) suggests: Understanding: Tell me the problem…tell me about the treatment Reason: What makes this treatment option better? Appreciation: Why do you think your doctor has recommended this treatment? Communication: Have you decided..? Can you tell me your decision?
Financial capacity	Tests of knowledge of income, assets, expenses, ability to write cheques and balance account statements, etc, as well as appreciation of how bills are paid, and consideration of financial problems and financial needs (Moberg & Pick, 2008). Can you tell me who you bank with and how much money you have in your accounts? Or how much goes in or out of your account on a regular basis? (Give patient coins/notes) Tell me which one is £1, £5, etc. If you're in a shop and you are buying a drink for X amount of money, what would you pay with and how much change would they give you? (Give patient change) Is this the right change? What would you do if you were not given the right change? If you had a budget of X for one month what would you spend it on? (Give patient a bill) Can you tell me how much the outstanding amount is? Are there any errors on the bill? (Give blank cheque) Can you fill out a cheque? (Consult with OT) Can patient use cash point, e.g. read words on screen and press correct buttons/talk to cashiers with aid if appropriate? What are the risks of not checking your bank statement regularly? What are the risks of not checking your change in a shop? What are the risks of not paying off your credit card? What are the risks of not paying your bills on time? What would you do if you lost your bank card/you noticed an error on your statement? Who could you ask for help? What are the risks of making purchases on the Internet? Why do you think these things would be difficult for you? Why do you think the team is concerned? Explain the team's concerns and recommendations and ask: Why do you think the team has recommended this?

Capacity to decide on discharge destination	What problems are you having right now?
	How do you think admission to a nursing home or home for the aged could help you with your condition?
	Can you think of other ways of looking after your condition?
	What could happen if you choose not to like living in a nursing home or home for the aged?
	What could happen to you if you choose to live in a nursing home or home for the aged?
	(These 5 questions are from the Ontario Ministry of Health and Long-term Care, 1997, cited by Carling-Rowland et al., 2014)
	What could be difficult when you go home?
	What do you have help with here in hospital?
	Who could you ask to help you?
	What are the risks of living on your own?
	What would happen if there were a fire/burglary, etc? (Ask patient to role play this if necessary)
	(Consult with OT/PT) Can patient use kitchen/bathroom, etc, safely? Can patient cook and clean independently? Can patient get to shops?
	What would you do if you fell over? (Consult with OT/PT) What are risks of falls in home? Can patient mobilise safely around the home?
	List some of the team's concerns and ask: Why do you think these things might be difficult for you?
	Explain the team's concerns and recommendations and ask: Why do you think the team has recommended this?

OT = Occupational Therapist, PT = Physiotherapist

Testamentary capacity and other areas

Moye et al. (2007) emphasise that other areas of decision-making, such as testamentary capacity, have received very little attention in the health literature to date. The following provides a brief summary of a couple of interesting and relevant areas to consider.

There are examples from as early as 1980 of SLTs supporting assessment of testamentary capacity (Ferguson et al., 2003 citing Udell et al., 1980). This may include conducting the assessment or supporting others to do this with communication tools such as the use of images and photos to demonstrate and communicate decisions. Ferguson et al. (2003) describe Enderby's (1994) recommendations for contributing to assessment of testamentary capacity, which include:

- assessing the individual's language, specifically: any disparity between their comprehension and expression;
- whether yes/no confusions occur;
- reading and writing skills;
- level of awareness of difficulties;
- attention;
- fatigue;
- emotional lability;
- perseveration.

Ferguson et al. (2003) go on to analyse a case study where the testamentary capacity of a lady with aphasia is challenged following her death. The researchers describe the lack of speech and language therapy assessment or expert advice in this case, yet the significance of the lady's communication difficulties. They flag the value that an SLT can add to domains such as understanding that she was making a will and what a will is, knowing who might legitimately expect to be left something in the will, knowing what she owned that could be left to others, and working out what to leave to whom.

Ferguson et al. (2003) emphasise the World Health Organisation's ICF framework and the SLT's role in social participation and, thus, the SLT's duty to their patients in facilitating their participation in legal responsibilities. The authors go on to make suggestions as to how to ensure that speech and language therapy assessments focus on functional abilities and strategies that can maximise performance when being used to complement capacity assessments. They also suggest videotaping the capacity assessments themselves, particularly in relation to testamentary capacity, as a means of providing evidence should the will later be appealed.

On a slightly different topic of capacity and competence, it is worth mentioning the little known area of registered intermediaries. Registered intermediaries were introduced by the Youth Justice and Criminal Evidence Act 1999, as one of the special measures available to help facilitate communication between the police, the courts and the vulnerable witness. Research has shown that this measure has been valuable in assisting the vulnerable witness to testify (O'Mahoney, 2010). The intermediary's role at investigative interview and trial is to enable 'complete, coherent and accurate' communication to take place. This includes facilitating communication, ensuring information is understood, and intervening when miscommunications occur (Plotnikoff & Woolfson, 2007). O'Mahoney (2010) collected information from intermediaries about their role and the 'needs' for vulnerable defendants requiring support. Of their sample, 58% were SLTs who all felt that intermediaries could have a positive role in supporting vulnerable defendants in their communication needs. Indeed, Plotnikoff and Wolfson (2007) report that the majority of registered intermediaries are SLTs.

Summary

Given the complexity of decision-making, the fact that there has been no single model of decision-making proposed as yet is perhaps not surprising (Gleichgerrcht et al., 2010). Many of us continue to make unwise decisions on a daily basis. Many of us do not make these wise or unwise decisions with complete capacity. We may make decisions without all the information, we may not wish to know or we may not have time to find out. Yet when one of our patients makes an unusual or unwise decision, or declines treatment, we question their decision-making capacity.

SLTs can advocate for a person's right to make their own wise or unwise decision in their own medical care, their finances or any other issue that may arise. Having a good understanding of how different cognitive issues can impact upon decision-making can assist us in this process. Each person we see, be they a person with aphasia, dementia, learning difficulties or a brain injury, will all have differing communication difficulties as well as differing values and beliefs. Morris et al. (2012) emphasise the overriding importance of assessing communication skills to understand a person's communication needs for decision-making. It can be particularly important in 'borderline' cases to understand the general functional abilities that may underlie the specific decision-making abilities and could lead to remediation of difficulties to ultimately enhance capacity.

Our patients' rights to communicate are a priority for us as SLTs. This should include their opinions or preferences about their care, their living circumstances, their finances, as well as what they would like to give to whom in their will. In fact, a significant part of our role in these areas of decision-making is to advocate for our patients' rights, and to break down barriers to this should they have the decision-making capacity to engage in this process. The next chapter discusses methods, communication aids and supports which may assist in this process.

References

Acquired Brain Injury and Mental Capacity Act Interest Group (2014) Acquired Brain Injury and Mental Capacity. Recommendations for Action following the House of Lords Select Committee Post-Legislative Scrutiny Report into the Mental Capacity Act: Making the Abstract Real.

Aldous, K., Tolmie, R., Worrall, L. & Ferguson, A. (2014) Speech-Language Pathologists' contributions to the assessment of decision-making capacity in aphasia: A survey of common practices. *International Journal of Speech-Language Pathology*, 16(3): 231–241.

Appelbaum, P. (2007) Assessment of patients' competence to consent to treatment. *New England Journal of Medicine*, 357: 1834–1840.

BBC Radio 4 (2015) Inside the Ethics Committee Series 11, episode 4: Withdrawing Feeding in Children

Bellhouse, J., Holland, A., Clare, I. & Gunn, M. (2001) Decision-making capacity in adults: Its assessment in clinical practice. *Advances in Psychiatric Treatment*, 7: 294–301.

Carling-Rowland, A., Black, S., McDonald, L. & Kagan, A. (2014) Increasing access to fair capacity evaluation for discharge decision-making for people with aphasia: A randomized controlled trial. *Aphasiology*, 28, 6: 750–765.

Cameron, L. & Murphy, J. (2006) Obtaining consent to participate in research: The issues involved in including people with a range of learning and communication disabilities. *British Journal of Learning Disabilities*, 35: 113–120.

Dickey, L., Kagan, A., Lindsay, M.P., Fang, J., Rowland, A. & Black, S. (2010) Incidence and profile of inpatient stroke-induced aphasia in Ontario, Canada. Arch.Phys.Med. Rehabil, 91(2): 196–202.

Dreer, L.E., Devivo, M.J., Novack, T.A., Krzywanski, S. & Marson, D.C. (2008) Cognitive predictors of medical decision-making capacity in traumatic brain injury. *Rehabil Psychol.* 1, 53(4): 486–497.

Dreer, L.E., Devivo, M.J., Novack, T.A. & Marson, D.C. (2012) Financial capacity following traumatic brain injury: A six month longitudinal study. *Rehabil Psychol.* 57(1): 5–12.

Ferguson, A., Worrall, L., McPhee, J., Buskell, R., Armstrong, E. & Togher, L. (2003) Case study: Testamentary capacity and aphasia: A descriptive case report with implications for clinical practice. *Aphasiology*, 17(10): 965–980.

Gleichgerrcht, E., Ibáñez, A., Roca, M., Torralva, T. & Manes, F. (2010) Decision-making cognition in neurodegenerative diseases. *Neurology.* 6: 611–623.

Goldbart, J. and Caton, S. (2010) *Communication and People with the Most Complex Needs: What Works and Why this is Essential*. London, Mencap.

Griffith, H.R., Belue, K., Sicola, A., Kryzywanski, S., Zamrini, E., Harrell, L. & Marson, D.C. (2003) Impaired financial abilities in mild cognitive impairment. A direct assessment approach. *Neurology*, 60(3): 449--457.

Heilbronner, R.L. (2011) Financial capacity. In: J. Kreutzer, J. DeLuca and B. Caplan (Eds) *Encyclopedia of Clinical Neuropsychology*, pp. 1047–1048. New York, Springer Science+Business Media.

Hoskin, K.M., Jackson, M. & Crowe, S.F. (2005) Can neuropsychological assessment predict capacity to manage personal finances? A comparison between brain impaired individuals with and without administrators. *Psychiatry, Psychology and Law*, 12(1): 56–67.

Hogden, A., Greenfield, D., Nugus, P. & Kiernan, M.C. (2012) Engaging in patient decision-making in multidisciplinary care for amyotrophic lateral sclerosis: The views of health professionals. *Patient Preference and Adherence*, 6, 691–701.

Hogden, A., Greenfield, D., Nugus, P. & Kiernan, M.C. (2013) What are the roles of carers in decision-making for amyotrophic lateral sclerosis multidisciplinary care? *Patient Preference and Adherence*, 7, 171–181.

Inglis, P. & Cook, T. (2011) Ten top tips for effectively involving people with a learning disability in research. *Journal of Learning Disabilities and Offending Behaviour*, 2(2): 96–104.

Jayes, M. & Palmer, R. (2013) Initial evaluation of the Consent Support Tool: A structured procedure to facilitate the inclusion and engagement of people with aphasia in the informed consent process. *International Journal of Speech-Language Pathology*, 1–10. DOI: 10.3109/17549507.2013.7959999

Jayes, M. & Palmer, R. (2014) Stroke research staff's experiences of seeking consent from people with communication difficulties: Results of a national online survey. *Topics in Stroke Rehab*. 21(5): 443–451.

Kagan, A. & Kimelman, M.K. (1995) Informed consent in aphasia research: Myth or reality. *Clinical Aphasiology*, 23, 65–75.

Kiani, R., Vahabzadeh, A., Hepplewhite, E.A., Abba, M., Finnamore, T., Bhaumik, S. & Satge, D. (2014) Overcoming challenges in diagnosing and treating cancers in people with intellectual disability: A case analysis. *Tizard Learning Disability Review*, 19, 51–58.

Kindell, J., Sage, K., & Cruice, M. (2015) Supporting communication in semantic dementia: Clinical consensus from expert practitioners. *Quality in Aging and Older Adults*, 16(3), 153–164.

Kleeberg, J., Bruggimann, L., Annoni, J.M., Melle, G.V., Bogousslavsky, J. & Schluep, M. (2004) Altered decision-making in multiple sclerosis: A sign of impaired emotional reactivity? *Ann Neurol*. 56: 787–795.

Knox, L., Douglas, J.M. & Bigby, C. (2015) 'The biggest thing is trying to live for two people': Spousal experiences of supporting decision-making participation for partners with TBI. *Brain Injury*, 29(6): 745–757.

Lo, B. (1990) Assessing decision-making capacity. *Law, Medicine and Health Care*, 18: 193–201.

Mackenzie, J.A., Lincoln, N.B. & Newby, G.J. (2008) Capacity to make a decision about discharge destination after stroke: A pilot study. *Clinical Rehabilitation*, 22: 1116–1126.

Marson, D.C. & Sabatino, C.P. (2012) Financial capacity in an aging society. *Generations, Journal of the American Society on Aging.* Blog entry http://www.asaging.org/blog/financial-capacity-aging-society-0

Marson, D.C., Stephen, J.D., Sawrie, M., Snyder, S., McInturff, B., Stalvey, T., Boothe, A., Aldridge, T., Chatterjee, A. & Harrell, L.E. (2000) Assessing financial capacity in patients with Alzheimer Disease. A conceptual model and prototype. *Instrument Arch Neurol.* 57(6): 877–884.

Marson, D.C., Dreer, L. E., Krzywanski, S., Huthwaite, J.S., DeVivo, M.J. & Novack, N.A. (2005) Impairment and partial recovery of medical decision-making capacity in traumatic brain injury: A 6-month longitudinal study. *Physical Medicine and Rehabilitation,* 86(5): 889–895.

Marson, D.C., Triebel, K. & Knight, A.(2012) Financial capacity. In G. Demakis (Ed.) *Civil Capacities in Clinical Neuropsychology. Research Findings and Practical Implications.* Oxford, Oxford University Press.

Martin, R., Triebel, K., Dreer, L., Novack, T., Turner, C. & Marson, D. (2012) Neurocognitive predictors of financial capacity in traumatic brain injury. *Journal of Head Trauma Rehabilitation,* 27(6): E81–E90.

McHugh, L. & Wood, R.L. (2008) Using a temporal discounting paradigm to measure decision-making and impulsivity following traumatic brain injury: A pilot study. *Brain Injury,* 22(9): 715–721.

Mental Capacity Act (2005) London, Department of Health. http://www.legislation.gov.uk/ukpga/2005/9/contents

Metz, D.E. & Folkins, J.W. (1985) Protection of human subjects in speech and hearing research. ASHA, 27: 25–29.

Moberg, P.J. & Pick, J.H. (2008) Decision-making capacity and competency in the elderly: A clinical and neuropsychological perspective. *Neurorehabilitation,* 23, 403–413.

Morris, R., Jones, J., Flew, R.J. & Mackenzie, J.A. (2012) Assessing mental capacity after a stroke: One year on. Presentation at the UK Stroke Forum, December 2012.

Moye, J., Karel, M.J.M., Azar, A.R. & Guerrera, R.J. (2004) Capacity to consent to treatment: Empirical comparison of three instruments in older adults with and without dementia. *The Gerentologist,* 44(2): 166–175.

Muhlert, N., Sethi, V., Cipolotti, L., Haroon, H., Parker, G.J.M., Yousry, T., Wheeler-Kingshott, C., Miller, D., Ron, M. & Chard, D. (2015) The grey matter correlates of impaired decision-making in multiple sclerosis. *J Neurol Neurosurg Psychiatry.* 86: 530–536.

Mukherjee, D. & McDonough, C. (2006) Clinician perspectives on decision-making capacity after acquired brain injury. *Topics in Stroke Rehabilitation,* 13(3): 75–83.

Murphy, J., Gray, C.M. & Cox, S. (2007) How 'Talking Mats' Can Help People with Dementia to Express Themselves: Full Report. Joseph Rowntree Foundation. www.jrf.org.uk. Downloaded from: http://www.jrf.org.uk/sites/files/jrf/2128-talking-mats-dementia.pdf

National Collaborating Centre for Mental Health commissioned by the Social Care Institute for Excellence National Institute for Health and Clinical Excellence (revised 2011) The NICE-SCIE Guideline on Supporting People with Dementia and their Carers in Health and Social Care. National Clinical Practice Guideline Number 42 published by The British Psychological Society and Gaskell. Downloaded from: http://www.nice.org.uk/nicemedia/live/10998/30320/30320.pdf

O'Mahoney, B. (2010) The emerging role of the Registered Intermediary with the vulnerable witness and offender: Facilitating communication with the police and members of the judiciary. *British Journal of Learning Disabilities*, 38(3): 232–237.

Owen, G.S., Frevenhagen, F. & Martin, W. (2015) Clinical assessment of decision-making capacity in acquired brain injury with personality change. *Neuropsychological Rehabilitation*, DOI: 10.1080/09602011.2015.1053948

Plotnikoff, J. & Woolfson, R. (2007) *The 'Go-Between': Evaluation of intermediary pathfinder projects.* Crown Copyright. ISBN 978 1 84099 080 5.

Royal College of Speech and Language Therapists (2005) Speech and Language Therapy Provision for People with Dementia. RCSLT Position Paper. London, RCSLT. Downloaded from: www.rcslt.org/resources/publications

Sachs, G.A. & Cassel, C.K. (1990) Biomedical research involving older human subjects. *Law, Medicine & Health Care*, 18(3): 234–243.

Simioni, S., Ruffieux, C., Kleeberg, J., et al. (2009) Progressive decline of decision-making performances during multiple sclerosis. *J Int Neuropsychol Soc.* 15: 291–95.

Skinner, R., Joiner, C., Chesters, L., Bates, L. & Scrivener, L. (2010) Demystifying the process? A multidisciplinary approach to assessing capacity for adults with a learning disability. *British Journal of Learning Disabilities*, 39: 92–97.

Stein, J. & Wagner, L.C.B. (2006) Is informed consent a "Yes or No" response? Enhancing the shared decision-making process for persons with aphasia. *Topics in Stroke Rehabilitation*, 13(4): 42–46.

Townend, E., Brady, M. & McLaughlan, K. (2007) Exclusion and inclusion criteria for people with aphasia in studies of depression following stroke: A systematic review and future recommendations. *Neuroepidemiology*, 29: 1–17.

Triebel, K.L., Martin, R.C., Novack, T.A., Dreer, L., Turner, C., Pritchard, P.R.,

Raman, R. & Marson, D.C. (2012) Treatment consent capacity in patients with traumatic brain injury across a range of injury severity. *Neurology.* 78(19): 1472–1478.

5 Assessing mental capacity as a speech and language therapist: Guidance and resources to improve practice

Mark Jayes

Introduction

There are a number of legal frameworks governing capacity across the UK, including the Mental Capacity Act (MCA, 2005). These describe in what circumstances a mental capacity assessment should be carried out, who is responsible for completing the assessment, and how capacity or incapacity should be determined. All these frameworks emphasise that, whenever a service user's ability to make an informed decision is in doubt, the professionals involved in that person's treatment or care (including the speech and language therapist, SLT) should consider carrying out a mental capacity assessment.

Mental capacity assessment findings can be contentious and emotive. The results impact directly on people's ability to retain independent control over many aspects of their lives (Lamont et al., 2013). The outcomes of capacity assessments can have significant long-term consequences for service users, their families and, in some cases, staff. Furthermore, assessment processes and conclusions may be examined by regulatory bodies such as the Care Quality Commission (CQC) and may be subject to legal scrutiny; a small but increasing number of legal cases are being brought to the Court of Protection by service users who wish to overturn the findings of capacity assessments. In short, it is important that assessments are compliant with the requirements of the relevant legal framework and provide accurate evaluations of service-users' decision-making ability.

Carrying out a high-quality assessment that is thorough and achieves an accurate judgement about decision-making ability is demanding. Assessors need to collect and consider a wide range of information in order to plan and carry out the assessment. They need to identify and use robust methods to test specific communicative and cognitive abilities underpinning decision-making capacity. Assessors need to be confident in these methods in order to justify and defend their conclusions about capacity. However, legal frameworks such as the MCA (2005) and its Code of Practice (2007) do not provide detailed instructions about the methods practitioners should use to assess capacity. In addition, there is no established gold standard mental capacity assessment tool available for staff to use. As a result, capacity assessment tends to be subjective (Ripley et al., 2008). This means that staff may find capacity assessment challenging and can lack confidence in their practice.

This chapter aims to clarify what a high-quality mental capacity assessment should include and how SLTs can prepare for and conduct this assessment. A number of assessment tools and communication aids that may facilitate and potentially improve capacity assessments are also discussed. Finally, relevant case studies are used to illustrate what forms the assessment process might take for service users presenting with different patterns of ability.

The assessment process

This section outlines a process for assessing mental capacity that is consistent with the requirements of the MCA (2005), the legislative framework in place in England and Wales. Elsewhere in the UK, the legal framework for Scotland is provided by the Adults with Incapacity (Scotland) Act (AISA, 2000), whilst in Northern Ireland a framework is proposed within the draft Mental Capacity Bill (MCB NI), which is still waiting to be presented to parliament. These three frameworks are based on similar principles relating to capacity and incapacity. They all describe processes that assessors should adopt in order to assess capacity and how assessors should form conclusions about whether or not a person has capacity. Although the required assessment processes are broadly similar across the different frameworks, there are some important differences. These differences will be discussed in relation to the specific aspects of the assessment process to which they relate.

What to consider before you start…

Is a formal capacity assessment required?

A capacity assessment is required when there is reason to believe an individual over the age of 16 years may lack the ability to make an informed decision for themselves. This could be because the person has a condition which may affect decision-making ability and has been found to lack capacity to make other decisions in the past. It may be because other people who know the person are concerned she or he may be unable to make a decision. Or it could be because the person's situation or behaviour causes people to question her or his capacity (MCA Code of Practice, 2007, paragraph 4.25).

It is worth noting that, even when there is strong reason to believe someone may not be able to make a decision for her or himself, a full formal capacity assessment is not indicated for every single decision. For example, an SLT who wishes to assess a person's communication or swallowing function needs to seek informed consent to do so. If the person is not able to give verbal consent, the therapist should take reasonable steps to check the person lacks capacity to consent and must be satisfied that the assessment is in the person's best interests before proceeding. Although the therapist does not need to document a formal process of capacity assessment, she or he would need to be able to describe what objective reasons led her or him to conclude the person lacked capacity to consent, if this judgement was later questioned (MCA Code of Practice, 2007, paragraph 4.44). Therefore, no formal assessment needs to take place for this decision. Other decisions, which may not require a full assessment, could include a service user deciding whether to receive personal care from a care worker or choosing which clothes to wear or what to eat for breakfast.

Is the assessment about a specific decision at a specific time?

A capacity assessment should only be used to determine an individual's ability to make a particular decision at the specific time it needs to be made. It should not be used to make judgements about general decision-making ability (MCA Code of Practice, 2007, paragraph 4.4). In a case brought to the Court of Protection, the Judge criticised a local authority for seeking a declaration that a woman with learning disabilities lacked capacity to make any decisions about daily living (*L v J* [2010] EWHC 2665 (Fam)). The Judge highlighted the need for separate capacity assessments to be initiated for individual decisions as they arose in the woman's life.

Thus, when preparing to carry out a capacity assessment, it is essential to consider exactly what decision the service user needs to make. If the decision appears to be made up of several sub-decisions, it is important to break this down and assess capacity for each individual decision. For example, sometimes SLTs are asked to contribute to assessments of a patient's ability to decide about 'discharge' from hospital. In reality, this may involve assessing whether the patient can decide if she or he wants to go home with or without support from carers. It may involve a decision about going home or going to live somewhere else where care can be provided (e.g. a residential or nursing home). This may lead to a decision about which facility in their local area the person wishes to choose, perhaps having visited a selection.

It is also important to confirm that the person needs to make the decision at this particular point in time. This is essential in cases where the person may have fluctuating capacity or a reversible condition that may affect capacity temporarily (e.g. due to an infection causing delirium). Whenever possible, the decision should be delayed until a time when the person may have regained capacity.

Who should assess?

Before the assessment process starts, it is important to identify the best person or people to carry out the capacity assessment. The assessor or assessors can be anyone "directly concerned" with the individual at the time the decision needs to be made (MCA Code of Practice, 2007, paragraph 4.38). However, the MCA Code of Practice also states that the "decision-maker", or person who ultimately makes a judgement about whether an individual has capacity to make the decision, should be the person who will take action in that individual's best interests if the assessment finds they lack capacity (MCA Code of Practice, 2007, paragraph 4.42).

Therefore, it usually makes sense for the decision-maker to assess capacity directly. This person is likely to understand the nature of the decision in question, the options available to the individual, and the consequences and associated risks and benefits of each option. Thus, medical staff are often involved in assessments about treatment decisions, whilst occupational therapists (OTs), discharge liaison nurses or social workers usually complete capacity assessments relating to care or residence decisions. As SLTs, we are often asked to carry out capacity assessments in relation to eating and drinking decisions for patients with dysphagia. Professionals with specialist financial or legal knowledge, sometimes social workers, are usually involved in capacity assessments relating to decisions about financial management, making a will or appointing a power of attorney.

In addition to understanding the nature of the decision and the options available to a service user, the capacity assessor needs to be able to discuss these options with the person and support her or him to understand and consider them. In order to do this effectively, the assessor should understand what might cause a person to have difficulty making a decision, and what support she or he may need to think about the decision and make a choice. The assessor may need to use specific skills or techniques to communicate with the person or to support her or his cognitive skills.

Certain disciplines are likely to have specialist knowledge and skills that will enable them to understand the needs of specific groups of patients during capacity assessments. For example, psychiatrists or other mental health professionals should understand how to approach assessments for people with mental health conditions. Similarly, psychologists and OTs are well placed to assess people with cognitive difficulties. As SLTs, we are ideally placed to assess capacity for a person with a communication disorder.

We may be asked to use our expertise in communication to facilitate our multidisciplinary colleagues' assessments of patients with communication disorders. We might carry out a specialist communication assessment and use our findings to advise colleagues how to support patients' individual communication needs during capacity assessments. Alternatively, we might participate in the capacity assessment in order to facilitate communication between the service user and the assessor and provide an opinion on the service user's ability to understand, retain and weigh information and communicate a decision. Alternatively, we may act as a joint assessor. It can be beneficial for two assessors with complementary knowledge and skills to carry out a joint assessment. Staff involved in mental capacity assessments have reported that they find joint assessments very useful, particularly in difficult cases where the judgement about capacity is not obvious and requires discussion with a colleague (Williams et al., 2012).

It appears that SLTs are involved to differing degrees and can play a number of roles in capacity assessment depending on established local patterns of practice. These issues are discussed further by Ferguson et al. (2010) and Suleman and Hopper (2015). In some settings, professional hierarchies appear to determine who assesses capacity (Shah et al., 2009a, 2010). It has been argued that SLTs should only ever play a facilitative role in capacity assessments and should not be the 'decision-maker' (Aldous et al., 2015). However, it could be argued that an SLT should be the decision-maker in a situation where the decision is whether or not to undergo a speech and language therapy investigation or intervention, for example a video fluoroscopy assessment; in these situations, the therapist or another SLT would be the person carrying out the endoscopy and would be well placed to make a judgement about the service user's best interests. Ultimately, the needs of the person being assessed and the nature of the decision should determine the choice of assessor.

How to approach the assessment

It is essential to remember the fundamental principles underpinning the relevant legislative framework when considering how to carry out a capacity assessment. Common to all UK legal frameworks is the need to assume the person being assessed has capacity to make the decision, unless it can be established through the process of assessment that she or he does not (e.g. MCA, 2005, section 1(2)). Within the UK legal frameworks, this assessment process needs to establish that the individual has some kind of disorder of the mind or brain, an inability to make the decision in question and that these two things are causally linked. For example, the MCA (2005) states that an individual may lack capacity if it can be established that she or he has an impairment or disturbance of the mind or brain that may affect her or his ability to make decisions (MCA, section 2(1)). Similarly, the AISA (2000) states that a person may lack capacity if she or he has difficulties making decisions "by reason of mental disorder or of inability to communicate because of physical disability or neurological impairment (AISA Short Guide, 2008, p. 9).

It should not be assumed that the individual lacks capacity merely because she or he has a certain condition (e.g. a diagnosis of dementia), appears to lack abilities associated with decision-making (e.g. communication or cognitive difficulties), or because she or he looks or behaves in a particular way (e.g. the person seems to make unwise decisions). In a case brought by service user 'K' to the Court of Protection, the Judge criticised previous capacity assessments relating to K's ability to make decisions about where to live on discharge from hospital (*CC v KK* [2012] EWHC 2136 (COP)). K, a woman with Parkinson's disease and vascular dementia, had wanted to return home but a number of assessments concluded she lacked capacity to make this decision; instead, she was discharged to a nursing home, which was considered to be in her best interests. The Judge suggested that the professionals who assessed K's capacity perceived her to be making an unwise decision, and that this influenced their finding of incapacity.

The two stage test

Stage 1: Identifying an impairment that affects decision-making

The first stage of the MCA two stage test requires assessors to establish whether or not the service user has an impairment or disturbance of the mind or brain which may affect the ability to make decisions (MCA (2005), section 2(1)). The Code of Practice (2007) provides examples of conditions that might cause such impairment or disturbance. These include temporary disturbances due to a delirium or alcohol use, and longer-term conditions due to neurological change (e.g. stroke, brain injury, progressive conditions such as Parkinson's disease or dementia), mental illness or learning disability. If no such impairment or disturbance is present, the assessor should conclude that the individual has intact capacity to make a decision.

Often the process of identifying and evidencing such an impairment or disturbance will be relatively straightforward. For example, the person may have an established diagnosis of a neurological or psychiatric condition that affects her or his cognitive and/or communicative function. The assessor may need to check the service-user's notes for a previous record of a diagnosis. Once the diagnosis is established, it can simply be documented as part of the capacity assessment. In some cases, however, the patient may not have a clear diagnosis. For example, this is often the case in situations where people have a degree of acute cognitive deficit or 'confusion' of uncertain origin, or a more chronic cognitive problem but have not been diagnosed with a neurological condition such as dementia. In these cases, the assessor should liaise with medical staff in order to establish a diagnosis. Alternatively, it may be possible to use cognitive, communication or psychiatric assessment findings as evidence of impairment. For example, a score on a cognitive screen such as the Montreal Cognitive Assessment (MoCA, Nasreddine et al., 2005) might be used to provide evidence of impairment of the functioning of the brain.

Stage 2: Assessing decision-making ability

If an impairment or disturbance is present, a functional assessment of the individual's decision-making ability should be conducted. Before the assessment takes place, it is important to take time to gather together all the information and resources needed to carry out a thorough assessment and consider various factors that could affect the service-user's responses during the assessment.

Preparing for the assessment

Gathering information about the decision

Firstly, the assessor needs a good understanding of the decision in question, in order to explain this adequately to the service user and assess her or his ability to make an informed decision. Case law suggests that capacity assessment findings can be overturned if it can be shown that assessors lack important knowledge about decisions. The case *PH and A local authority and Z unlimited* [2011] EWHC 1704 (Fam) involved legal scrutiny of a capacity assessment for a man with Huntington's disease who wished to leave a specialist care unit in order to return to his own home. The Judge said the assessment was invalid because the assessor had not been aware of all the man's care needs.

Key information to establish before the assessment should include:

- What decision options are available to the service user?

- Why does the decision need to be made now?

- What are the known benefits and risks associated with each option?

- What are the likely consequences of the service user choosing each option or of not making a decision at all?

Gathering information about the service user

Next, the assessor needs to identify any cultural, ethnic or religious factors that may impact on the service user's decision-making process and should be considered when planning the assessment. For example, it would be important to establish whether a service user might respond to treatment options in certain ways because of her or his religious beliefs. It would be essential to consider this type of information when making a judgement about a person's ability to weigh and use information in order to make a decision, especially if the person's beliefs conflicted with those of the capacity assessor.

Similarly, it would be important to consider whether cultural attitudes to decision-making may affect a service-user's responses during a capacity assessment. In some cultures, decisions may usually be taken jointly with other members of the community (Morris, 2012). In such cases, it might be beneficial to involve others in the assessment process. It would also be important to ascertain if the service user has made any advance decisions that are relevant to the current decision. For example, the service user may have made an advance decision not to receive any alternative nutrition or hydration in certain circumstances.

The assessor needs to establish if the service user has any communication, cognitive or mental health needs which may affect the assessment process, and how these needs might best be met in order to support the individual's decision-making abilities. Communication needs might relate to level of alertness, visual or hearing deficits, speech or language impairments, or to the service user not being a native speaker. Information about these needs and potential methods for supporting them might be found in the service user's notes or in a communication passport or history form, or by talking to the service user, her or his family and friends or other people working with the service user. If a difficulty is suspected but confirmatory information is not available, a referral should be made to the relevant specialist service for an assessment (e.g. hearing or vision services or an interpreting service). As SLTs, we have a key role in identifying communication difficulties and providing information to other staff about people's communication needs and how they can be supported. Our role is to identify inclusive communication methods to use within the capacity assessment to support the service user's understanding and expressive communication skills. Inclusive communication approaches are discussed in the next section.

Cognitive needs might relate to level of alertness, orientation, memory, attention or executive function difficulties. All of these difficulties can impact directly on decision-making ability. Again, information about these needs and ways to support them may be available in the service user's notes or from the service user, family or friends, or other staff. In some settings, SLTs may be involved in assessing cognitive functions. Alternatively, a referral should be made for specialist cognitive assessment by a psychologist or occupational therapist or other discipline, depending on local practice. This can be particularly valuable because certain cognitive difficulties (especially those relating to executive function) may be very subtle and difficult to detect using standardised assessments (Herbert, 2013). Suleman and Kim (2015) provide a useful overview of the relationship between cognitive skills and decision-making. It is always important not to conflate performance on cognitive assessments with decision-making ability in order to draw conclusions about a person's mental capacity, as the two are not the same (Morris, 2012).

Mental health conditions might affect a service user's cognitive and communication skills, which would impact on decision-making ability. Relevant conditions include mood disorders such as depression or bipolar disorder and schizophrenia. Some SLTs may have specialist skills in working with this population. For other SLTs, it would be important to liaise with mental health specialists (e.g. a psychologist, community psychiatric nurse or psychiatrist) in order to establish how the condition may affect the individual's mental capacity and how to support her or him during a capacity assessment. Doing a joint assessment with other specialist professions, such as a psychiatrist or OT, can ensure the service user's decision-making abilities are fully recognised.

Facilitating communication: The key role of the speech and language therapist

All the UK legal frameworks for assessment of mental capacity require assessors to provide practical support in order to maximise service users' ability to make decisions, before it can be established that they lack capacity. As mentioned in Chapters 2 and 3 of this book, useful information about these issues is provided by chapter three of the MCA Code of Practice (2007) and a guidance document (Scottish Government, 2008) relating to the Adults with Incapacity (Scotland) Act 2000. The MCA (2005) requires assessors to provide information "in a way that is appropriate to (the service user's) circumstances" in situations where service users may have difficulty understanding language (MCA, 2005, paragraph 3(2)). Chapter 3 of the MCA Code of Practice (2007) provides useful but very broad guidance about how assessors might support people to understand information relating to a decision, for example:

> "Information must be tailored to an individual's needs and abilities. It must also be in the easiest and most appropriate form of communication for the person concerned." (Mental Capacity Act Code of Practice, 2007, p. 31)

The chapter suggests ways that information can be adapted in order to make it more accessible, for example by using simple language and relevant pictures or objects to communicate ideas.

For patients with difficulties using language to express their thoughts or choices, both the MCA and AISA Codes of Practice recommend that provision is made to enable them to use alternative communication methods to express themselves. The MCA Code of Practice (2007) also suggests potential methods that might be used to support people with speech or expressive language difficulties to communicate their understanding, opinions and choices. These include picture boards, sign and symbol systems, and computer-based technology.

However, the Codes of Practice do not provide guidance on how to identify the methods to use to meet service users' individual needs. They do emphasise the importance of referring to speech and language therapy for specialist support in this complex area. As SLTs, we need to use our knowledge of the evidence base, clinical experience and practical skills to create information materials and strategies that are tailored to the individual communication needs and preferences of each service user. Our key role within mental capacity assessment is emphasised within the RCSLT "Five Good Communication Standards" document (RCSLT, 2013) and in the RCSLT's submission to the public consultation on proposals for the Draft Mental Capacity Bill in Northern Ireland (2014).

The first part of the SLT's role is to carry out a thorough assessment of the service user's communication needs and preferences.

What a communication assessment needs to include

The assessment should start with a detailed case history. It is important for the therapist to gain information on existing effective and preferred communication methods from the service user and anyone else who knows her or him well (family, friends and relevant professionals). The assessment needs to examine the service user's speech and all four modalities of language use: spoken understanding, reading, use of spoken language and writing. It is essential to establish if the service user has a reliable "yes/no" response and whether anything can be done to facilitate this. The aim of this assessment is to identify relative strengths and needs which can then be used to identify appropriate support methods to use during the capacity assessment. Case study 1 below provides a practical example of how an SLT's communication assessment contributes to the preparation of a capacity assessment.

The assessment can involve both formal and informal methods. The therapist may wish to start with a screening assessment in order to identify specific areas of functioning to assess in more detail using more specialist assessments. Examples of tools that can be used to assess speech and language for the purposes of planning capacity assessments are listed below in Table 5.1. In some settings, SLTs may be involved in assessing cognitive function. In these situations, the therapist can make use of a number of formal assessment tools to identify cognitive strengths and needs. Examples of cognitive assessments are also shown in Table 5.1. Again, the purpose of any cognitive assessment would be to identify the most effective ways to support the service user's needs during the capacity assessment, in order to maximise her decision-making ability.

Table 5.1 Examples of assessment tools that can be used to plan capacity assessments.

Domain of function	Clinical population	Assessment tool
General communication (screening assessments)	Adults with communication difficulties	Stirling Understanding Screening Tool (SUST) (Cameron & Murphy, unpublished)
	Adults with aphasia	Frenchay Aphasia Screening Test (FAST) (Enderby et al., 2012) Consent Support Tool (available in Jayes & Palmer, 2014)
Language modalities	Adults with acquired language disorders	Test for Reception of Grammar (TROG-2) (Bishop, 2003)
	Adults with aphasia	Comprehensive Aphasia Test (CAT) (Swinburn et al., 2005) Reading Comprehension Battery for Aphasia (RCBA-2) (LaPointe & Horner, 1998)
	Adults with dementia	Arizona Battery for Communication Disorders of Dementia (ABCD) (Bayles & Tomoeda, 1993)
	Older adults	Barnes Language Assessment (Bryan et al., 2001)
Cognitive-language functions	Adults with traumatic brain injury	Measure of Cognitive-Linguistic Abilities (MCLA) (Ellmo, 1995) Mount Wilga High Level Language Test (Simpson, 2006)
	Adults with neurological impairment due to stroke, head injury or dementia	Cognitive Linguistic Quick Test (CLQT) (Helm-Estabrooks, 2001)
Cognitive functions (general)	Adults with cognitive difficulties (check whether test is standardised for use with a specific clinical population)	Addenbrooke's Cognitive Examination III (ACE-III) (Hsieh et al., 2013) Montreal Cognitive Assessment (MoCA) (Nasreddine et al., 2005)

Case Study 1: Preparing an assessment

Mr J is admitted to hospital for a planned surgical procedure. Staff notice that following surgery, Mr J appears confused and he is diagnosed with post-operative delirium. The medical team decide that the delirium is caused by an infection and recommend that Mr J has further surgery to manage the infection. Mr J's medical consultant visits him on the ward to discuss the surgery and she finds that Mr J appears very distracted and his responses to her questions about the surgery make her doubt that he has understood what she has said to him. The consultant is concerned that Mr J may lack capacity to consent to the surgery and decides she needs to carry out a capacity assessment. Unfortunately, the decision about surgery cannot be delayed, so the assessment needs to be completed promptly. The consultant refers Mr J to speech and language therapy for an assessment of his communication skills, so that she can gain more information to help plan the capacity assessment.

The SLT takes a thorough case history for Mr J from his medical notes and also talks to other members of the multidisciplinary team to gain further information about his communication and cognitive function. Other staff have observed that Mr J can be distractible and sometimes does not appear to understand what people say to him. They say he seems to manage better in the mornings when he is not too tired. Staff report they are able to understand Mr J when he talks to them.

The SLT assesses Mr J's communication informally at bedside. She considers using the Cognitive Linguistic Quick Test (CLQT, Helm-Estabrooks, 2001) to establish whether Mr J has cognitive difficulties which may impact on his communication skills and his decision-making ability. However, Mr J is very distracted and becomes agitated early on during the communication assessment, so she decides not to use the formal assessment. The communication assessment indicates that Mr J can answer questions containing up to two information carrying words reliably, using spoken "yes" and "no" responses. He can understand sentences with up to three information carrying words when he is able to concentrate better on what the therapist is saying. It helps Mr J to pay attention when the therapist draws the curtains around the bed and says Mr J's name at the start of sentences.

The assessment shows that the content of Mr J's expressive language is sometimes tangential and repetitive but he does not have any significant word-finding difficulties. It helps Mr J to keep to the topic of conversation when the therapist reminds him what they are talking about. It also helps when she writes down words and sentences corresponding to the topic of conversation and points to them.

The SLT documents her assessment findings in the medical notes and uses them to draw up a list of recommended ways for staff to maximise Mr J's communication and attention skills. She places one copy of these in Mr J's notes and another at his bedside. She talks to the ward team about these recommendations. The consultant feels the recommendations will help her to plan her capacity assessment but is concerned she may need help communicating with Mr J. Therefore, she asks the therapist to attend the capacity assessment in order to ensure that Mr J's communication skills are fully supported.

The therapist and consultant decide to carry out the capacity assessment in the morning at a quieter time on the ward, when Mr J may concentrate better. They would like to assess Mr J in a quiet side room but this is not possible. Instead, they plan to close the curtains around Mr J's bed and ensure there is not too much noise in the bay (they will ask for the TV to be turned off). They invite Mr J's daughter to attend the assessment, as staff on the ward have noticed that Mr J appears calmer when she is with him. The SLT and consultant discuss what information Mr J needs to be told about his operation and how they will explain this. The therapist prepares some cards with keywords and sentences in simple language that can be used to explain information to Mr J and help him to pay attention and keep on track with the conversation. The therapist also prepares cards with simple language questions that can be used to check Mr J's ability to understand, retain and weigh up the information he is given.

Identifying effective methods to facilitate communication

As SLTs, we are trained to identify and use different methods to support people to understand information and express themselves. The draft RCSLT Position Paper on 'inclusive communication' provides more information about ways to support people's communication (RCSLT, 2015). This document uses the term 'inclusive communication' as an umbrella term to describe all approaches to supporting people to understand information and express themselves, including total communication, augmentative and alternative communication (AAC) methods and accessible information techniques.

Total communication involves the use of any verbal or nonverbal communication method that may support people to maximise their ability to communicate. Total communication methods include speech and writing, any type of vocalisation, use of images (including line drawings, photographs, symbol systems, cartoons and video), objects and physical actions (including gesture, pointing at things, facial expression and mime) (Rautakoski, 2011). These methods can be used by the individual with the communication difficulty and those communicating with her or him.

Like the total communication approach, augmentative and alternative communication (AAC) methods involve the use of different verbal and nonverbal methods to supplement or replace speech and language (Beukelman & Mirenda, 2005). AAC may be unaided and involve the use of total communication methods (e.g. sign systems, gesture, facial expression). Alternatively, AAC may involve low-tech aids such as individualised communication books or alphabet charts, or high-tech electronic aids (e.g. involving speech generating devices or computer software).

An example of a low-tech AAC system is Talking Mats© (see Figure 5.1). This system involves simple picture symbols which can be placed along visual scales in order to support people to understand information and express feelings, preferences, needs and choices in relation to different topics. The system has been used by people with learning disabilities (Murphy & Cameron, 2008), motor neurone disease (Murphy, 1999), dementia (Murphy & Oliver, 2013) and aphasia (Murphy, 2000). More information about Talking Mats© is available at http://www.talkingmats.com/

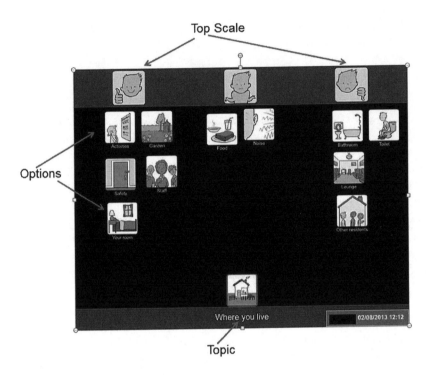

Figure 5.1 Example of how Talking Mats© can be used to support people in expressing their decisions. This Talking Mat shows how a woman with dementia feels about where she lives:

- She is happy with activities, garden, safety, staff, own room
- She is unsure about snacks and noise
- She is unhappy about bathroom, toilet, lounge and other residents.

Submats could be used to explore some of these issues in more detail (reproduced by permission of J. Murphy, www.talkingmats.com).

Another very useful AAC resource (illustrated in Figure 5.2) has been specifically developed by two UK SLTs to assist healthcare professionals to support the needs of hospital patients with communication difficulties during capacity assessments (Allen & Bryer, 2014). This set of materials includes general guidance about capacity assessment, specific information about working with patients with communication disorders, and a set of photographs and diagrams that can be used to support conversations about a range of common decisions during capacity assessments. It can be accessed at http://www.blacksheeppress. co.uk/products/adults/MCA.

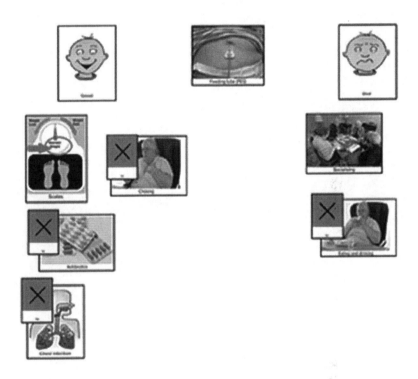

Figure 5.2 Example of how the *Supporting Adults with Communication Impairment to make Decisions* resource can be used in discussions about non-oral feeding options (Copyright Heart of England NHS Foundation Trust 2014, with permission).

In Canada, Carling-Rowland (2012) has developed the Communication Aid to Capacity Evaluation (CACE). This AAC resource provides a capacity assessment process for staff to use with people who have aphasia, motor speech disorders or hearing loss and also with people who speak English as a second language. The resource has been specifically designed for assessments involving decisions about whether to go to live in a nursing or residential home. It includes a text- and image-based booklet that can be personalised and used to structure a conversation with the person about her or his decision, using supported conversation techniques. The CACE and its training video are available at: http://www.aphasia.ca/home-page/health-care-professionals/resources-and-tools/cace/

The term 'accessible information' can be interpreted in different ways. A useful definition sees it as information that is presented in such a way that it can be understood and used easily by its target audience (Litherland, 2007). There are a number of guidelines that SLTs can use to make information more accessible. These guidelines tend to relate to the use of simplified language and other visual methods (e.g. images) to make text-based information easier to read and understand. A summary of guidelines that are relevant to people with communication disorders associated with different conditions is provided in Table 5.2.

Table 5.2 Guidelines for making written information accessible to different clinical populations.

Clinical population	Producing organisation	Name of guidance document
People with hearing and visual difficulties	Social Care Institute for Excellence (SCIE)	How to produce information in an accessible way (SCIE, 2005) Available at: http://www.scie.org.uk/
People who have had a stroke	Connect – The Communication Disability Network	Including people with communication disability in stroke research and consultation: A guide for researchers and service providers (Connect, 2007)
	Stroke Association	Accessible Information Guidelines (Stroke Association, 2012) Available at: https://www.stroke.org.uk/shop/product/accessible-information-guidelines
	University of Queensland	Four key aphasia-friendly principles for adapting written information (described by Brennan et al., 2005, p. 695)
	National Institute for Health Research (NIHR) Clinical Research Network: Stroke	Engaging with people who have aphasia: a set of resources for stroke researchers (NIHR, 2014) Available at: http://www.crn.nihr.ac.uk/blog/news/new-aphasia-resources-for-researchers-conducting-stroke-studies/

People with learning disabilities	Change/National Equality Partnership	How to make information accessible: A guide to producing easy read documents (CHANGE/National Equality Partnership 2009) Available at: http://www.changepeople.org/free-resources/
	Department of Health (DH)	Making written information easier to understand for people with learning disabilities (DH, 2010). Available at: https://www.gov.uk/government/publications/making-written-information-easier-to-understand-for-people-with-learning-disabilities-guidance-for-people-who-commission-or-produce-easy-read-information-revised-edition-2010
	Mencap	Make it Clear (Mencap, 2009) Available at: https://www.mencap.org.uk/make_it_clear
	Social Care Institute for Excellence (SCIE)	How to produce information in an accessible way (SCIE, 2005) Available at: http://www.scie.org.uk/
People who have had a brain injury	Headway	Coping with communication problems after brain injury (Headway, 2014) Available at: https://www.headway.org.uk/shop.aspx
People with dementia	Dementia Engagement and Empowerment Project (DEEP)	Writing dementia-friendly information (DEEP, 2013). Available at: http://dementiavoices.org.uk/wp-content/uploads/2013/11/DEEP-Guide-Writing-dementia-friendly-information.pdf

Most of these guidance documents were created by experts working in collaboration with people with communication difficulties. The guidance makes recommendations for adapting the content and design of information materials in order to increase their accessibility. These recommendations tend to be broadly consistent across the different clinical populations. They are summarised in Table 5.3.

Table 5.3 Common content and design principles for making written information accessible to people with communication disorders.

Use simple, everyday words and sentence structures.

Use short sentences with one main idea per sentence.

Use clear photographs to illustrate important single concepts.

Use communication symbols if the reader is familiar with them.

Use a sans serif font of at least size 14 point.

Highlight important information using bold, headings and text boxes.

Break up text using line spacing, bullet points, headings and white space.

Involve the target audience in the creation of adapted information.

It is essential to trial any total communication strategies or accessible information materials with a service user before using them within a capacity assessment, for three reasons. First, it is important to establish that these methods actually help the individual to communicate more effectively. Because service users present with different patterns and severities of communication difficulty, they will require different types of support to help them understand and some may still be unlikely to benefit from support.

There is some research evidence relating to which types of people are likely to benefit most from these systems. For example, research on the effectiveness of Talking Mats© to support people with learning disabilities suggests the system may be most effective for people who are able to understand at least three information carrying words (Murphy & Cameron, 2008). Research involving the use of Talking Mats© by people with dementia suggests that the system can help people at different stages of the dementia process and their family carers to feel more involved in discussions that include decision-making, and more satisfied with the outcomes of these discussions (Murphy & Oliver, 2013). Research within the aphasia literature suggests that simplifying language, highlighting key information and using large, clear text fonts and extra spacing may help people with mild-to-moderate comprehension difficulties to understand more information but may not benefit those with more severe difficulties (Jayes & Palmer, 2014; Brennan et al., 2005; Rose et al., 2003). However, the effectiveness of many inclusive communication methods has not been widely researched. Therefore, it is important to always trial these methods with service users in order to check whether they are actually of help.

Second, it is important to ascertain whether a service user is willing to use the communication method or strategy. Some people may be reluctant to use certain methods, even those that appear to help them. For example, research suggests some people with aphasia may not appreciate the use of pictures because they find them patronising or childish (e.g. Rose et al., 2012). Third, it is important to verify that the individual can use these methods functionally. For example, it would be important to ascertain whether a person was able to recognise and extract meaning from images before creating visual resources to use within the capacity assessment. This could be checked informally, by asking the individual to select the image from other distractor images, in response to a verbal instruction, description or question, or by asking them to match different images from a single semantic category. There are more formal methods for assessing the ability to use images meaningfully, for example the Multimodal Communication Screening Test for Persons with Aphasia (MCST-A, Garrett & Lasker, 2007). Similarly, it would be important to verify the service user was able to use gesture or drawing functionally to support understanding and expression before introducing these methods to the capacity assessment. Furthermore, it would be beneficial to practise using inclusive methods before a capacity assessment, in order to maximise an individual's ability to use them during the assessment. Case study 2 below illustrates some of these issues.

Case Study 2: Facilitating expression

Mr V has Progressive Supranuclear Palsy and has been admitted to hospital because he has fallen and fractured his hip. Mr V has fallen a number of times before at home and hospital staff and Mr V's family are concerned he is at risk of further falls. He now needs to make a decision about his living and care arrangements on discharge from hospital. A capacity assessment has been initiated by the multidisciplinary team because members of Mr V's family and some ward staff have concerns that Mr V may have difficulty making a decision because his communication and cognitive abilities have been affected by his neurological condition and the effects of his acute illness. The speech and language therapy team has been asked to carry out a joint capacity assessment with Mr V's OT.

An SLT prepares for the capacity assessment by checking whether Mr V has been seen by speech and language therapy before. The therapist finds out that Mr V was seen at home by colleagues in the community speech and language therapy team for assessment and management of his speech and swallowing difficulties. Before admission to hospital, Mr V had mild dysarthria but was usually able to use some intelligibility strategies to communicate well. The SLT visits Mr V on the ward to carry out a communication assessment. This involves taking a detailed case history from Mr V's medical notes, from ward staff and from Mr V himself. She assesses Mr V's communication skills using an informal screening tool. This shows that Mr V is able to understand complex spoken sentences, understand well in conversation and is able to recall the content of a conversation over the course of the assessment. Mr V's dysarthria is now severe and he is no longer able to use intelligibility strategies to increase the clarity of his speech.

The therapist assesses Mr V's reading and writing ability to identify any total communication strategies that could be used to help him express himself during the capacity assessment (e.g. writing things down, pointing to written words). Mr V can read written paragraphs and answer yes/no questions about their content accurately. Unfortunately, Mr V cannot write because he has extremely limited arm and hand movement, due to muscle weakness. The therapist investigates whether Mr V can use his eyes to point to words or pictures to help him express himself. Mr V is able to point to single words and pictures and is able to use an E-tran frame to spell out short words. Mr V also appears interested in using the E-tran frame again to have conversations with his family and ward staff.

Based on the assessment, the SLT hypothesises that Mr V should be able to understand a spoken explanation about the discharge decision during the capacity assessment if the explanation is given in lay language. Mr V will need support during the assessment to ask and answer questions and express his opinions. The E-tran frame appears to be an effective, low-tech AAC device to use to facilitate this and Mr V appears happy to use it. To maximise Mr V's ability to use the frame during the capacity assessment, the SLT recommends that Mr V, his family and ward staff practise using the frame during conversations on the ward. This works well and Mr V becomes a proficient user of the frame. The mental capacity assessment takes place three days later. The OT and SLT use lay language to explain the various living arrangement options to Mr V and the benefits and drawbacks of each. They ask him questions to check his understanding and to ascertain which option he prefers and why this is so. Mr V uses the E-tran frame to explain to the therapists what he understands about his situation, where he would like to live and why this is the case.

Other practical considerations

There are a number of additional practical issues to address in order to ensure the service user is given the best opportunity to demonstrate her or his decision-making ability. These relate to when and where the assessment takes place and who attends. The assessment should be scheduled at a time when the service user is likely to be most alert, most relaxed and least distracted. Care should be taken to incorporate sufficient breaks to ensure the person does not become too tired or distracted. It should take place in a confidential environment that supports the person's communication and cognitive skills and makes her or him feel relaxed and comfortable. Usually, this will be somewhere quiet with few visual or audible distractions and it could be in a familiar setting that is reassuring to the service user; it could also be in a setting that is relevant to the decision that needs to be made in order to provide additional contextual information that may help to make the decision-making process less abstract for the service user. For example, a service user living in the community, who needs to make a decision about going into hospital for treatment, might benefit from being given information related to the treatment in a hospital setting.

It is important to ensure the service user has access to any equipment that supports her or his communication needs, for example working hearing aids, a hearing loop system, clean glasses, a pen and paper, or any other communication aids. Additional support may be provided by inviting relevant people to attend the assessment. These could be professionals who can offer specialist support with cognitive or mental health needs, professionals who have specialist knowledge relating to the decision that needs to be made, or a family member, friend or other person (e.g. familiar carer) who may be able to support the service user's needs (including communication) and whose presence may be reassuring. It is important to explain in advance to these people why the capacity assessment needs to take place, what it will involve, and what their role is likely to be. Bear in mind that family members or friends may hold specific views about the service user's level of ability, including her/

his mental capacity, and may wish to make you aware of this; this could make the assessment process challenging at times.

How to structure the assessment itself

The MCA and AISA Codes of Practice do not prescribe how capacity assessments should be structured, how long they should be, how formal or informal they should be, or exactly what information or questions they should include. This is because each assessment will be unique and will depend on the individual natures of the decision and the service user's circumstances and support needs.

Currently there is little published evidence describing how people carry out capacity assessments. The available research evidence and descriptions in case law reports suggest a common approach is to use a semi-structured conversation format to deliver information about decisions and assess service users' decision-making abilities (e.g. Emmett et al., 2013). In this approach, the assessor engages the service user in a conversation about the decision. This conversation might take place in one session, or may need to be spread over a number of sessions, depending on the service user's ability to participate without fatiguing. Capacity assessment is often a dynamic process involving multiple assessment sessions and various discussions with staff, the service user and her or his family or friends. When sufficient time is available, perhaps in a rehabilitation or community setting, this process may involve a targeted approach to educate the service user about the decision and use therapeutic techniques to enhance her or his ability to understand, retain, weigh information and communicate a decision.

In certain circumstances, taking more time to complete the assessment may be challenging, especially if there is pressure to make a decision quickly (for example, in an acute hospital setting when the decision is about discharge arrangements). However, the MCA Code of Practice (2007) warns against rushing assessments and there is legal precedent that could be used to justify devoting enough time to carry out thorough assessments. In the case *PH and A local authority and Z unlimited* [2011] EWHC 1704 (Fam), the Judge questioned the validity of the assessment, stating that at only 90 minutes long, it is likely to have been superficial. Herbert (2013) argues that the time allotted to capacity assessment should depend on how urgently the decision needs to be made, but should also be commensurate with the significance and complexity of the decision and its consequences.

Although the exact structure or format of each assessment will vary, the vital components should always be the same. The assessment needs to enable the assessor to: i) verify that the service user has been given all the information she or he needs to make a decision, in whatever way supports the service user to understand and think about the decision; ii) make a judgement about the service user's decision-making ability (according to the requirements of the local legal framework); iii) ascertain the service user's views about the decision and her or his preferred option, in order to inform future planning.

What information to give the service user

The main types of information that should be explained to the service user during the assessment include:

- What the decision is
- Why the decision needs to be made now
- The different decision options
- The associated risks and benefits for each option
- The likely consequences of choosing each option or of not making the decision
- How the decision may affect the service user and people around them.

The MCA Code of Practice (2007) explains that it is important to strike a balance between giving the service user enough information to help her or him to make a decision and including too much detail, which may be confusing. Even though information may be simplified in order to make it easier to understand, it is essential that it includes all the salient information the service user needs, including the full range of options available to her or him. In the legal case *CC v KK* [2012] EWHC 2136 (COP), the Judge overturned a previous judgement that K lacked capacity to make a decision about where to live on leaving hospital because the Judge concluded that K had not been given detailed information about her care options and was therefore not in a position to be able to weigh them up in order to make an informed decision.

Which abilities to test during the assessment

The different legal frameworks operating across the UK define the abilities that need to be assessed in order to make a judgement about a person's capacity. All the UK frameworks require an assessment of the service user's ability to: i) understand information related to the decision to be made; ii) retain that information for the purposes of making the decision; iii) use or weigh the information; iv) communicate a decision using any means. However, the law in Scotland and the proposed bill for Northern Ireland require additional assessments relating to the abilities to remember and weigh up information for the purposes of decision-making. This information is summarised in Table 5.4.

Methods for testing each ability

Any capacity assessment needs to provide evidence that the assessor has tested the different abilities underpinning decision-making in a robust way. Otherwise, the validity of the judgement about capacity will be questionable. Again, the MCA and AISA Codes of Practice do not specify methods for testing understanding, retention and weighing of information or communication of a decision. An obvious way to check these abilities is simply to use a semi-

Table 5.4 Summary of UK legal requirements for what to include in tests of decision-making ability.

Assessment domain	Requirements of each UK legal framework		
	MCA (2005)	AISA (2000)	MCB NI (proposed)
Comprehension	Ability to understand information related to the decision. NB: in order to demonstrate capacity, the person being assessed needs to understand information that is most relevant to the decision, but not every detail of the information provided.		
Memory	Ability to retain that information for as long as it takes to make the decision (i.e. may only be for a short period).	Ability to retain that information long enough to be able to make the decision and act on it.	Ability to retain that information for as long as it takes to make the decision.
Executive function skills	Ability to use or weigh that information in order to make a decision.	Ability to use or weigh that information in order to make a decision and act on it.	Ability to use or weigh that information and appreciate its relevance.
Expressive communication	Ability to communicate a decision using any means.		

structured conversation format to ask the service user questions about the decision, the options available, her or his preferred choice and why she or he has reached this decision.

However, this approach is unlikely to support all the needs of service users with any degree of communicative or cognitive difficulty. This aspect of capacity assessment is challenging. However, as previously mentioned, due to our training and experience, we SLTs are well placed to identify and implement novel methods for testing understanding and for supporting people to express their opinions and choices. These methods are likely to involve use of total communication strategies, AAC and accessible information formats to enable the assessor to ask questions that are accessible to the service user and to support the service user to respond and express her or his opinions. The choice of method will depend on the individual's profile of communication strengths and needs, which will be informed by the communication assessment carried out in preparation of the capacity assessment. Table 5.5 suggests methods that could be used to test the abilities associated with decision-making capacity of people with communication difficulties. The Scottish Government document *Communication and Assessing Capacity: A guide for social work and health care staff* (2008) provides other useful methods and guidance.

Table 5.5 Methods for testing the abilities underpinning decision-making for use with people with communication needs

Ability to be tested	Suggested methods
Understanding the information	Ask person to say/write down what she or he has understood about the decision, the need for a decision, the options available and potential consequences of these.
	Encourage the person to use total communication methods to communicate what she or he has understood (e.g. gesture, drawing).
	Present forced alternatives (e.g. "Am I talking about an operation or a tablet?").
	Ask "yes/no" questions (e.g. "Am I talking about an operation?").
	Ask the person to select written words or phrases corresponding to important concepts from distractors.
	Ask the person to select visual images corresponding to important concepts from distractors (e.g. using Talking Mats©, Allen & Bryer (2014) images or other symbol system).
	Ask the same question using different methods or ensure questions are phrased in different ways, in order to check consistency of responses (e.g. "Is the decision about [correct answer]?", "So you need to make a decision about [incorrect answer]?").

Retaining the information	Use the same methods as for understanding.
	Check consistency of responses throughout assessment.
	Check the consistency of responses at later points in time, if legal framework requires this (e.g. AISA, 2000).
Weighing or using the information to make a decision	Ask the person to say/write down why she or he has chosen a particular option.
	Encourage the person to use total communication methods to communicate why she or he has chosen a particular option (e.g. gesture, drawing, pointing to images).
	Ask the person to say/write down the pros and cons of options.
	Ask the person to select written words or phrases corresponding to pros/cons, risks or benefits of options.
	Ask the person to select visual images corresponding to pros/cons, risks or benefits (e.g. using Talking Mats©; Allen & Bryer (2014) images or other symbol system).
	Encourage the person to use total communication methods to communicate what she or he would do in a particular situation (e.g. if she or he fell over at home; if there was a fire in the house).
	Present forced alternatives (e.g. "Which is safer, going home or staying here?").
	Ask "yes/no" questions (e.g. "Could drinking water make you ill?");
Communicating a decision	Encourage person to use intelligibility strategies or AAC if they have a motor speech difficulty.
	Encourage person to use total communication methods (e.g. an alphabet chart).
	Ask "yes/no" questions ("Do you want to…?").

Making a decision about whether a service user has demonstrated each ability sufficiently in order to make an informed decision is very challenging. Often assessors report that, if they are in any doubt, they find it helpful to ask a colleague for a second opinion. Joint assessment can be beneficial, as it gives assessors the opportunity to share observations of the service user. It is important to remember that a key principle of the MCA (2005) is to assume the person being assessed has capacity to make the decision, unless the assessor can show on the 'balance of probabilities' that they do not. This means the assessor needs to be satisfied and be able to evidence that it is more likely than not that the person lacks capacity at that time to make that decision. In Case study 3, the SLT makes a judgement about the service user Ms C's capacity to make a decision about what types of drinks she has, based on his observation that it is more likely than not that she does not understand the risks involved in drinking unthickened drinks. Chapter 4 of the MCA Code of Practice (2007) provides useful information about these issues.

Whenever we make a decision about a service user's capacity it is important to consider whether the person's circumstances mean that we should review this decision at a future date. This is especially important in cases when a service user has fluctuating capacity (for example associated with a temporary condition such as a delirium) but the decision they need to make cannot be delayed. It would also be important to review someone's capacity if we expected her or his decision-making ability either to deteriorate due to a degenerative condition or improve due to recovery in health status or neurological function.

When a capacity assessment concludes that a person lacks capacity to make a decision, it is still important to try to involve her or him in the decision-making process. If a best interests decision-making process is initiated, then this should include consideration of which decision option the service user prefers, if she or he has been able to communicate this during or outside the capacity assessment. It is also crucial to share information with the service user, whenever possible, about the outcomes of assessments, discussions and meetings related to the decision in question, in order to facilitate her or his understanding of what is happening and inclusion in the process. This may help staff to maintain or even restore a trusting relationship with the service user, who may have been unhappy about the outcome of the capacity assessment.

Case Study 3: Being facilitator and decision-maker

Ms C had a stroke several years ago that left her with communication and swallowing difficulties. She has aphasia which affects her understanding and ability to express herself verbally. She and her partner use total communication strategies to overcome these difficulties. These strategies were introduced by the community speech and language team that last saw Ms C and her partner a few years ago. Ms C has been having fork-mashable texture food for many years and manages this well. However, her partner has noticed that Ms C has been coughing a lot recently whenever she has a cup of tea. She has also had a chest infection in the last month. Ms C's GP visits her and is concerned her dysphagia may have worsened. Therefore, the GP refers her for a swallow assessment.

The assessment indicates that Ms C is at risk of aspirating drinks but that the risk is reduced if she has her drinks thickened. When the therapist explains this, Ms C reacts badly and makes it clear that she does not want to have her drinks thickened. The therapist discusses this with Ms C's GP and they decide that it would be beneficial to assess Ms C's capacity to make a decision about her drinks in order to satisfy themselves that she is making an informed decision. They think she may lack capacity because they are not convinced she really understands the risks associated with drinking, because of her aphasia.

The SLT agrees to carry out the capacity assessment and prepares by carrying out a thorough communication assessment. This involves taking a detailed case history from Ms C and her partner, from Ms C's GP and her previous speech and language therapy notes. Next, the therapist assesses Ms C using the Comprehensive Aphasia Test (CAT, Swinburn et al., 2005). This shows that she can understand spoken single words and some short sentences but cannot reliably understand longer sentences involving more complex grammar. Ms C has moderate word-finding difficulties that limit her ability to express herself in conversation. However, during the assessment, she spontaneously uses gesture and drawing to help get her message across. She also finds a communication book that she made with her previous SLT and points to a photograph of an object in the book to answer a question on the language assessment. The therapist tries using these strategies in conversation with Ms C and notes that they appear to support her understanding as well as her expression. The language assessment indicates that Ms C is able to read some high frequency single words but cannot read sentences reliably. It also shows that she is no longer able to spell words accurately, due to dysgraphia.

Based on what he has observed during the assessment, the SLT hypothesises that Ms C will have difficulty understanding spoken or written explanations about her swallowing difficulties during the capacity assessment and will need support to express her understanding of these difficulties and her reasons for not wanting to have her drinks thickened.

The therapist decides to use simple spoken language together with total communication methods, such as gesture, drawing and pointing to images and objects, to explain to Carol about her dysphagia and the options available to her.

He decides that he will encourage Carol to use the same methods to respond to his questions, when he checks how much she understands and what she thinks about her dysphagia. With Carol's agreement, the therapist invites Dave to be present during the assessment, as Dave will be able to offer reassurance to Carol and may be able to support her communication skills. They decide to hold the assessment in the morning because Dave has noticed that Carol communicates best at this time.

Before the assessment, the therapist plans which resources he will need to use during the capacity assessment. These include blank sheets of paper, pens, diagrams of the muscles involved in swallowing, a tin of thickening powder and a prepared thickened drink. The therapist plans the methods that he will use to ask Carol specific questions during the assessment. He considers how to ask these questions using simplified language, and designs a rating scale using images and simple words to enable Carol to express her preferences. He tests out this rating scale before the assessment by asking Carol to point to the scale to indicate if she likes certain TV programmes. Dave is able to confirm that Carol's responses appear reliable.

During the assessment, Carol is able to use total communication strategies to demonstrate that she understands she has a swallowing difficulty but her responses to the questions indicate that she does not understand that these swallowing difficulties may cause her to have chest infections. The therapist repeats this information a number of times using different communication methods, but Carol is not able to demonstrate that she understands the risks associated with continuing to have unthickened drinks. The therapist concludes that, on the balance of probabilities, Carol lacks capacity to make an informed decision about what type of drinks she should have. Dave agrees with this conclusion. The therapist documents this in Carol's electronic speech and language therapy notes, which the GP can also access. The therapist and GP start to plan a best interests meeting with Dave and Carol.

Documentation

Judgements made by care providers about a service user's ability to make day-to-day decisions (e.g. about what to wear or have for breakfast) or give consent to receiving care do not require recorded documentation (MCA Code of Practice (2007), paragraph 4.60). However, all formal capacity assessments require accurate and comprehensive documentation. A contemporaneous and unambiguous record of the assessment will help other people working with the service user to understand and act on the findings of the assessment. It will also provide evidence that the assessor has followed the principles of the relevant legal framework should the assessment findings ever be scrutinised or challenged.

The MCA Code of Practice (2007) suggests that capacity assessments should be documented in professional records, which may include a person's medical notes or a care plan, depending on the assessment context. Where and how the assessment is recorded will also depend on local policy and relevant professional standards. For example, SLTs should comply with RCSLT record keeping standards. This is currently provided in section 5.5.3 of Communicating Quality 3 (RCSLT, 2006) but this document is being revised.

The UK legal frameworks do not specify exactly what types of information assessors should include in their records of capacity assessments. In order to be able to use the record to justify a conclusion reached about a person's capacity, it is suggested that the record should include the following information:

- Who were present during the assessment and what their roles were

- The nature of the decision the service user was asked to make

- The salient information the service user needed to understand about the decision

- The evidence gathered relating to the presence/absence of an impairment or disturbance of the mind or brain and, if present, whether it was temporary or permanent[*]

- How the abilities underpinning decision-making capacity were assessed[*]

- What support was provided to help the service user to make the decision

- The evidence collected relating to the service user's ability to understand, retain and weigh information about the decision and communicate her/his decision[*]

- If the person lacked one these abilities, how this was related to an impairment or disturbance of the mind or brain
- The assessor's conclusion about the service user's capacity to make that decision
- If the service user was judged to have capacity, what decision she or he made
- If the service user was judged to lack capacity, whether she or he was able to indicate a preference for a particular decision option
- The management plan (e.g. to plan a best interests meeting/refer to an advanced decision/consult a nominated attorney/review capacity at a later date).

* depending on the requirements of the legal framework

A documentation aid such as a proforma may facilitate record keeping. As well as providing a means for the assessor to document her or his observations during the capacity assessment and conclusions about the service user's capacity, proformas can be designed to remind the assessor what the assessment should include, in order for it to comply with the legal framework. An example of such a proforma is provided below.

Tools to facilitate assessment

A number of tools have been developed to support people to carry out mental capacity assessments. Some of these tools have been designed specifically to facilitate and increase the reliability of assessment of capacity to consent to treatment or to participate in research studies. Lamont et al. (2013) and Sturman (2005) have reviewed these tools and summarised evidence about their usefulness. The majority of the tools involve structured or semi-structured interview formats that enable assessors to structure their capacity assessments and document their observations. Several tools provide structures to facilitate the assessment of the ability to understand, retain and weigh up information and communicate a choice.

In his review, Sturman (2005) identified the MacArthur Competence Assessment Tool-Treatment (MacCAT-T, Grisso et al., 1997) as the 'gold standard' tool for assessing capacity to make decisions about treatment options. This tool supports the assessor to provide personalised information

Mental Capacity Assessment Process Proforma (Mark Jayes & Rebecca Palmer, 2014)

Name of person being assessed:
Name of assessor: Date of assessment:

Decision to be made

Q: What is the decision? _____

Is it a single, specific decision?   YES → Continue   NO → Stop: review decision, break it down
Does decision need to be taken now?   YES → Continue   NO → Stop: start again when decision required

Mental capacity assessment: Stage 1

Q: Does the person have an impairment of the mind or brain, or a disturbance* affecting the way the mind or brain works?

YES (on balance of probabilities) → Continue   NO → Stop: Assume person has capacity to make decision

Evidence (e.g., diagnosis / evidence of communication or cognitive deficits): _____
_____

*If temporary disturbance (e.g., delirium), could decision be delayed until disturbance resolved?

Mental capacity assessment: Stage 2

Functional test of decision-making ability: Does that impairment or disturbance mean that the person is unable to make the decision in question at the time it needs to be made?

Consider: Are you the best person to assess decision-making?
Do you know the individual and their situation?
Are you able to support their communication and cognition?
Could somebody else help?

> If unsure, recruit help from MDT / carers / family / friends

Consider: Have you gathered all the necessary information for the assessment?
What options are available to the person?
What are the consequences / benefits / risks of each option?
Are there any cultural / ethnic / religious factors to consider?
What are the person's communication and cognitive needs?
How can you best support these needs? (strategies, resources, interpreters)

> If unsure, consult notes / MDT / carers / family / friends

Consider: Best time of day/ environment for assessment, including carer/family/friends.
Check: Person has clean glasses / working hearing aids.

Q: Does the person have a general understanding of what decision they need to make and why they need to make it?

YES (on balance of probabilities) → Continue   NO → Stop: Person lacks capacity to make decision

Evidence:_____
_____
_____
_____
_____

1

Mental Capacity Assessment Process Proforma (Mark Jayes & Rebecca Palmer, 2014)

Name of person being assessed:
Name of assessor: **Date of assessment:**

Q: Does the person have a general understanding of the likely consequences of making, or not making, this decision? (they need to understand all salient information relating to the decision)

   YES (on balance of probabilities) → **Continue**   **NO** → **Stop:** Person lacks capacity to make decision

Evidence:_____

_____

_____

_____

Q: Is the person able to retain information relevant to the decision <u>long enough to make the decision</u>?

   YES (on balance of probabilities) → **Continue**   **NO** → **Stop:** Person lacks capacity to make decision

Evidence:_____

_____

_____

_____

Q: Is the person able to weigh up all information relevant to the decision?

   YES (on balance of probabilities) → **Continue**   **NO** → **Stop:** Person lacks capacity to make decision

Evidence:_____

_____

_____

_____

Q: Is the person able to communicate their decision <u>by whatever means possible</u>?

YES (on balance of probabilities) → Person has capacity to make decision

NO → Person lacks capacity to make decision

Evidence:_____

_____

_____

_____

Conclusion of assessment

Q: Does person have capacity to make this decision?

      YES   **NO** → **Plan Best interests Meeting**

<u>**Now place proforma / document this process in person's medical records / care plan**</u>

to the service user about the medical condition that requires treatment, the treatment options available to her or him, and the associated risks, benefits and likely consequences of these options. The tool also prompts the assessor to ask questions that examine the service user's understanding and appreciation of this information and their reasoning about the decision. Lamont et al. (2013) concluded that the MacCAT-T had been well tested across different clinical populations, including medical inpatients and people with dementia, cognitive impairment and mental health conditions. It is important to note that tools like the MacCAT-T are designed primarily to help assessors collect information and think about decision-making capacity rather than provide determinations of people's capacity; their use cannot replace clinical judgement about capacity and does not guarantee compliance with UK capacity law.

A number of tools or processes have been developed specifically for use with people with communication needs. As noted above, Allen and Bryer (2014) have produced a resource pack to facilitate capacity assessments for hospital patients with communication difficulties. The pack contains guidance about planning the capacity assessment and assessing communication skills, provides downloadable AAC materials and techniques for using these, and also includes documentation aids. Oldreive and Waight (2011) have developed a structured assessment pathway for assessing the capacity of people with learning disability to decide whether to sign a tenancy agreement. This assessment pathway includes language and literacy screening assessments which can be used to adapt information about the tenancy decision to make it more accessible to service users' individual needs. The pathway also includes processes for assessing a service user's reasoning and money skills, to inform a judgement about her or his capacity to make the decision.

Similarly, Skinner et al. (2011) have developed a capacity assessment algorithm for multidisciplinary staff to use with people with learning disability who need to make decisions about having eye surgery. The algorithm prompts staff to consider various factors that may impact on capacity, including communication and memory skills and mental health status. The algorithm provides a mechanism for screening communication ability that enables staff to decide when to refer to speech and language therapy for specialist support.

The Consent Support Tool (described in Jayes & Palmer, 2014) was designed to enable stroke researchers to identify research participants with communication needs and provide information in accessible ways during the informed consent process. It includes a language screening test and suggests methods for tailoring written information to make it more accessible to individual needs. Although designed specifically to help researchers support people with aphasia or motor speech disorders to make decisions about taking part in research studies, this tool could be adapted for use with people with other communication disorders who need to make a range of decisions. For example, it could be used to adapt written information about decisions to meet the needs of individuals with cognitive-communication disorders secondary to brain injury or neuro-degenerative conditions, such as dementia or Multiple Sclerosis.

Finally, a number of audit tools have been developed to help assessors reflect on their capacity assessments and evaluate their quality. The Assessment of Mental Capacity Audit Tool (AMCAT, Mental Health Foundation, 2015) provides an online learning resource and audit tool. The tool asks multiple-choice questions about the assessment process, including the rationale for assessing, the type of person being assessed, how the assessment was planned and carried out, how the person was supported and what the outcome was. The tool is meant to take 20 minutes to complete and generates a report summarising and commenting on the information that the assessor has inputted. This can be used as a learning tool to support reflective practice. The audit tool is available at http://www.amcat.org.uk/

The British Psychological Society's (BPS) Audit Tool for Mental Capacity Assessments (2010) provides a set of detailed quality standards that can be used to measure assessment quality. The standards relate to different aspects of the assessment: preparatory information gathering; assessment of specific abilities; methods used to enhance capacity or facilitate decision-making; documentation; recommendations for future actions. The standards were based on information contained within the MCA (2005) and its Code of Practice (2007), RCSLT and College of Occupational Therapists professional guidelines, published research and from medico-legal sources. This audit tool is designed to help improve practice at both individual practitioner and service or team levels. It is available online at: http://www.bps.org.uk/sites/default/files/documents/audit-tool-mental-capacity-assessments_0.pdf

Summary

Mental capacity assessment is a growing area of health and social care practice. Capacity assessment is challenging and brings with it significant responsibility. It involves a careful balance between promoting people's right to autonomy and protecting them from harm. Inaccurate assessment places service users at risk, either of being excluded from decision-making when it is wrongly concluded they cannot make decisions, or of making uninformed decisions when it is incorrectly judged that they can. Assessments are increasingly subject to scrutiny by regulatory bodies and the judicial system. Therefore, it is important that assessors prepare their assessments thoroughly and provide information about decisions in ways that support service users' individual needs. Assessors need to use robust methods to assess the different information-processing abilities underpinning decision-making capacity. Assessment documentation needs to include unambiguous, comprehensive information about these methods, assessment findings and management plans. A number of tools have been developed to facilitate these activities but more resources are needed.

As SLTs, we are experts in assessing and supporting communication skills. This means we are ideally placed to play a key role in capacity assessment. We have an important role in providing specialist assessment and identifying and implementing facilitative communication methods to support the needs of people with communication disorders during the assessment process. We also have a responsibility to educate our multidisciplinary colleagues about the role of communication in decision-making, in order to support them to improve their assessment practice. Importantly, we should always apply the principles of evidence-based practice whenever we engage in mental capacity assessment, in order to ensure we use the most effective methods we can to support people with communication needs to engage in decision-making.

Resources

Information about legislative frameworks for capacity assessment

Lay summary of the Mental Capacity Act (2005) for service users and families: https://www.gov.uk/government/uploads/system/uploads/attachment_data/file/365631/making_decisions-opg601.pdf

Mental Capacity Act (2005) Code of Practice (2007): https://www.gov.uk/government/publications/mental-capacity-act-code-of-practice

Adults with Incapacity (Scotland) Act 2000: A short guide to the Act: http://www.gov.scot/Publications/2008/03/25120154/0

Adults with Incapacity (Scotland) Act Code of Practice (3rd edition, 2010): www.gov.scot/Resource/Doc/327864/0105906.pdf

Adults with Incapacity (Scotland) Act 2000. Communication and Assessing Capacity: A guide for social work and health care staff http://www.gov.scot/Publications/2008/02/01151101/12

UK mental capacity legal summaries and case law reviews: http://www.mentalcapacitylawandpolicy.org.uk/

RCSLT Response to NI Mental Capacity Bill 2014 consultation (discusses role of speech and language therapists in capacity assessment): http://www.rcslt.org/governments/docs/draft_mentalcapacity_bill

Practical tools to aid capacity assessment

Visual resources and guidance for supporting hospital patients during capacity assessments by Allen & Bryer (2014): http://www.blacksheeppress.co.uk/products/adults/MCA#

Assessment of Mental Capacity Audit Tool: http://www.amcat.org.uk/

British Psychological Society guidance on good practice and assessment audit tool: http://www.bps.org.uk/sites/default/files/documents/audit-tool-mental-capacity-assessments_0.pdf

RCSLT Inclusive information resources http://www.rcslt.org/members/professional_standards/inclusive_communication/inclusive_communication

Total communication information and resources: http://totalcommunication.org.uk

NHS England Information Standard: http://www.england.nhs.uk/tis/

Social Care Institute for Excellence guidance on accessible information: http://www.scie.org.uk/publications/misc/accessguidelinespublications.asp

Talking Mats information and resources: http://www.talkingmats.com/

Royal College of Speech and Language Therapists (RCSLT) Five good communication standards: http://www.rcslt.org/news/docs/good_comm_standards

Alzheimer's Society information on cognitive assessment of people with dementia: https://www.alzheimers.org.uk/cognitiveassessment

This chapter is based on independent research arising from a Clinical Doctoral Research Fellowship supported by the National Institute for Health Research (NIHR) and Health Education England (HEE).

Any views expressed in this chapter are those of the author and not necessarily those of the NHS, the NIHR, the HEE or the Department of Health.

References

Aldous, K. et al. (2015) Speech-language pathologists' contribution to the assessment of decision-making capacity in aphasia: A survey of common practices. *International Journal of Speech-Language Pathology*, 16: 231–241.

Allen, J. & Bryer, H. (2014) Supporting Adults with Communication Impairment to Make Decisions. Available from: http://www.blacksheeppress.co.uk/products/adults/MCA#

Bayles, K.A. & Tomoeda, C.K. (1993) *Arizona Battery for Communication Disorders of Dementia (ABCD)*. Austin TX, PRO-ED.

Beukelman, D.R. & Mirenda P. (2005) *Augmentative and Alternative Communication: Supporting Children and Adults with Complex Communication Needs,* 3rd ed. Baltimore MA, Paul H. Brookes Publishing Co.

Bishop, D'& Worrall, L. (2010) Legal decision-making by people with aphasia: Critical incidents for speech pathologists. *International Journal of Language and Communication Disorders,* 45(2): 244–268.

Garrett, K.L. & Lasker, J.P (2007) *The Multimodal Communication Screening Test for Persons with Aphasia (MCST-A).* Available from: http://cehs.unl.edu/aac/aphasia-assessment-materials/

Grisso, T., Appelbaum, P.S. & Hill-Fotouhi, C. (1997) The MacCAT-T: A clinical tool to assess patients' capacities to make treatment decisions. *Psychiatric Services,* 48: 1415–1419.

Headway (2014) *Coping with Communication Problems after Brain Injury.* Nottingham, Headway – the brain injury association.

Helm-Estabrooks, N. (2001) *Cognitive Linguistic Quick Test (CLQT).* San Antonio TX, Pearson Education Inc..

Herbert, C. (2013) Mental capacity In: L.H. Goldstein and J.E. McNeil (Eds) *Clinical Neuropsychology: A Practical Guide to Assessment and Management for Clinicians,* 2nd edition, pp. 445–459. Chichester, John Wiley & Sons.

Hsieh, S. et al. (2013) Validation of the Addenbrooke's Cognitive Examination-III in Frontotemporal Dementia and Alzheimer's Disease. *Dementia and Geriatric Cognitive Disorders,* 36(3–4), 242–50. Test available from: www.neura.edu.au/frontier/research/test-downloads.

Jayes, M. & Palmer, R. (2014) Initial evaluation of the Consent Support Tool: A structured procedure to facilitate the inclusion and engagement of people with aphasia in the informed consent process. *International Journal of Speech-Language Pathology,* 16(2): 159–168.

Lamont, S., Jeon, Y-H. & Chiarella, M. (2013) Assessing patient capacity to consent to treatment: An integrative review of instruments and tools. *Journal of Clinical Nursing,* 22(17–18): 2387–403.

LaPointe, L.L. & Horner, J. (1998) *Reading Comprehension Battery for Aphasia (RCBA-2).* Austin TX, PRO-ED.

Litherland, R. (2007) Developing the resources people with dementia need. *Journal of Dementia Care,* 15(6): 15–17.

Mencap (2009) *Make it Clear.* Available at: https://www.mencap.org.uk/make_it_clear

Mental Health Foundation (2015) *Assessment of Mental Capacity Audit Tool (AMCAT).* Available at: http://www.amcat.org.uk/

Morris, R. (2012). Decision making and mental capacity. In: N. Lincoln, (Ed.) *Psychological Management of Stroke,* pp. 203-231. Oxford: Wiley-Blackwell.

Murphy, J. (1999) Enabling people with motor neurone disease to discuss their quality of life. *Communication Matters Journal,* 13(2): 2–6.

Murphy, J. (2000) Enabling people with aphasia to discuss quality of life. *British Journal of Therapy and Rehabilitation*, 7(11): 454–457.

Murphy, J. & Cameron, L. (2008) The effectiveness of Talking Mats for people with intellectual disability. *British Journal of Learning Disability*, 36: 232–241.

Murphy, J. & Oliver, T.M. (2013) The use of Talking Mats to support people with dementia and their carers to make decisions together. *Health & Social Care in the Community*, 21(2): 171–180.

Nasreddine, Z.S. et al. (2005) The Montreal Cognitive Assessment, MoCA: A brief screening tool for mild cognitive impairment. *Journal of the American Geriatrics Society*, 53(4): 695–699.

National Institute for Health Research Clinical Research Network: Stroke (2014) *Engaging with People who have Aphasia: A Set of Resources for Stroke Researchers.* Available from: http://www.crn.nihr.ac.uk/blog/news/new-aphasia-resources-for-researchers-conducting-stroke-studies/

Office of Public Sector Information (2005) *Mental Capacity Act 2005.* London, OPSI.

Oldreive, W. & Waight, M. (2011) Assessment of capacity: Reflections from practice. *Learning Disability Practice*, 14: 31–36.

Rautakoski, P. (2011) Training total communication. *Aphasiology*, 25(3): 344–365.

Ripley, S., Jones, S. & Macdonald, A. (2008) Capacity assessments on medical in-patients referred to social workers for care home placement. *The Psychiatrist*, 32: 56–59.

Rose, T.A. et al. (2012) Guiding principles for printed education materials: Design preferences of people with aphasia. *International Journal of Speech-Language Pathology*, 14(1): 11–23.

Rose, T., Worrall, L. & McKenna, K. (2003) The effectiveness of aphasia-friendly principles for printed health education materials for people with aphasia following stroke. *Aphasiology*, 17(10): 947–963.

Royal College of Speech and Language Therapists (RCSLT) (2006) *Communicating Quality 3: RCSLT's Guidance on Best Practice in Service Organisation and Provision.* London, RCSLT.

Royal College of Speech and Language Therapists (RCSLT) (2015) *Draft Position Paper: Inclusive Communication.* London, RCSLT.

Shah, A., Banner, N/, Newbigging, K., Heginbotham, C. & Fulfrd B (2009a) The early experience of consultant psychiatrists in application of the Mental Capacity Act: Issues for black and minority individuals. *Ethnicity and Inequality in Health and Social Care*, 2: 4–10.

Shah, A., Banner, N., Heginbotham, C. & Fulford, B. (2009b) The application of the Mental Capacity Act 2005 among geriatric psychiatry patients: A pilot study. *International Psychogeriatrics,* 21: 922–930.

Shah, A., Banner, N., Heginbotham, C. & Fulford, . (2010) The early experience of old age psychiatrists in the application of the Mental Capacity Act 2005: A pilot study. *International Psychogeriatrics*, 22, 147–157.

Simpson, F. (2006) *Mount Wilga High Level Language Test (Revised edition 1)*. Available from: http://www.aphasiafriendly.co/Free_Resource_Library_2.html

Skinner, R. (2011) Demystifying the process? A multidisciplinary approach to assessing capacity for adults with a learning disability. *British Journal of Learning Disabilities*, 39: 92–97.

Social Care Institute for Excellence (2005) *How to Produce Information in an Accessible Way*. Available from: http://www.scie.org.uk/publications/misc/accessguidelinespublications.asp

Stroke Association (2012) *Accessible Information Guidelines*. Available from: http://www.stroke.org.uk/sites/default/files/Accessible%20Information%20Guidelines.pdf.pdf

Sturman, E.D. (2005) The capacity to consent to treatment and research: A review of standardized assessment tools. *Clinical Psychology Review*, 25: 954–974.

Suleman, S. & Hopper, T. (2015) Decision-making capacity and aphasia: Speech-language pathologists' perspectives. *Aphasiology*. DOI: 10.1080/02687038.2015.1065468

Suleman, S. & Kim, E. (2015) Decision-making, cognition, and aphasia: Developing a foundation for future discussions and inquiry. *Aphasiology*. DOI: 10.1080/02687038.2012.1049584

Swinburn, K., Porter, G. & Howard, D. (2005) *The Comprehensive Aphasia Test*. Hove, UK: Psychology Press.

The British Psychological Society (BPS) (2010) *Audit Tool for Mental Capacity Assessments*. Leicester, The British Psychological Society.

The Scottish Government (2008) *Adults with Incapacity (Scotland) Act 2000*. Edinburgh, The Scottish Government.

The Scottish Government (2008) *Adults with Incapacity (Scotland) Act 2000: A short guide to the Act*. Edinburgh, The Scottish Government.

The Scottish Government (2010) *Adults with Incapacity (Scotland) Act 2000 Code of Practice (Third Edition)*. Edinburgh, The Scottish Government.

Williams, V. et al. (2012) *Making Best Interests Decisions: People and processes* [online]. London, Mental Health Foundation. Available from: http://www.mentalhealth.org.uk/content/assets/PDF/publications/BIDS_report_24-02-12_FINAL1.pdf?view=Standard [Accessed 29 June 2012].

6 Roles and relationships in the multidisciplinary team when assessing mental capacity

Hannah Luff and Anna Volkmer

Introduction

Speech and language therapists (SLTs) have a unique set of skills to offer to the process of assessments of decision-making capacity. Working within the multidisciplinary team (MDT) is a crucial part of this. When it comes to matters of capacity and best interests decisions, the MDT is likely to include a variety of professionals from within health and social care. This team may also include wider members of the community, such as police, solicitors, people working in finance and housing officers. Thus it is important that each individual's role is clearly defined, including the limitations of this role. This will ensure clarity on what each member of the team offers from the outset. We will discuss the challenges of this later in the chapter.

There are more likely to be divisions within the team when there is a complex decision to be made and the 'best interests' of the individual are unclear. This is when personal values and prejudices may be most evident. It is important in these situations that people are aware of their own values and how this affects their overall judgement. Individuals will be more or less risk adverse and influenced by their views and experiences.

Where decision-making capacity is in doubt, an effective MDT must share the responsibility for gathering evidence to support or refute capacity. An individual may perform poorly in a formal test, but demonstrate sound judgement in a more practical situation. The team should be committed to clarifying decision-making capacity. If a person does not have decision-making capacity the team should endeavour to work with the individual and family members or other representatives, such as Independent Mental Capacity Advocates (IMCAs), to arrive at a suitable course of action.

The Mental Capacity Act (MCA) Code of Practice (2007) recommends that capacity assessments be conducted in pairs. This approach will increase the rigour and robustness of the assessment, which in turn should increase accuracy and reduce bias in the assessment process.

Role of the SLT in the assessment of capacity

The SLT may have a number of different roles within the assessment of capacity, some of which may overlap. Time resources are usually limited, and there can be a tension between time spent on these areas and time spent on other speech and language therapy activities. There are no easy answers to this question, but prioritising risks appropriately and being clear about what will have the most impact for that individual is a useful starting point (see Chapter 1).

Where it seems likely that a capacity assessment and any ongoing communication support and decision-making is going to be time-consuming, it is useful to make a plan which covers the key areas that the professional is going to address and which are outside their remit. Regardless of timing, being clear with the team you are working with about the roles you will each take in a particular meeting or episode of care will provide clarity and reduce misunderstandings.

Flew and Holly (2011) advocate that SLTs have a number of different roles to play in assessing a person's capacity.

The SLT as assessor

An SLT may be involved in directly assessing the decision-making capacity of a person (Volkmer, 2013). This may arise in numerous dysphagia-related issues, but particularly where an SLT may have recommended alternative feeding. In these situations, the SLT may be one of the key professionals involved in conducting the capacity assessment itself. In fact, there may be many situations where we are doing these types of assessments. When a person has known communication impairments, it is not always clear on first meeting what modifications are required and the act of starting an assessment in and of itself requires agreement from the person. Thus many sessions may commence with a type of capacity assessment.

The SLT as advocate

In a situation where it is difficult for a person to express their wishes without a support, the SLT may act as an advocate. In some situations, it may be preferable that the SLT should not also give an opinion on the individual's capacity, as it may represent a conflict of interests. Acting as an advocate is different from acting as an 'aid to communication'.

Acting as an advocate for a person can arise after the SLT has spent time interacting with the person with communication difficulties, for example in individual therapy sessions, where the person's views and opinions have come to light. This information can then be shared with the MDT. At times, this may be more of an 'impression' than a concrete statement made by the person, and the SLT needs to make it clear that this is the case. This type of information should be considered as subjective evidence in any decision-making. These 'impressions' are more open to interpretation and personal biases and, while they can provide a valuable patient perspective, should be treated with caution.

The SLT as educator or advisor

The SLT is uniquely placed to engage in a range of formal and informal assessments to establish communication abilities and limitations, in addition to looking at how nonverbal strategies can help the individual to express his or her wishes (Jayes & Palmer, 2013). This may be to help support a specific decision, or to provide more general information to the MDT and others to communicate with an individual. The role here may end with providing a written summary of communication to support the person in all situations or may require the SLT to go on to provide training to others (Carling-Rowland et al., 2014).

The SLT as aid to communication

The second statutory principle of the MCA (2005) states that:

> "A person is not to be treated as unable to make a decision unless all practicable steps to help him to do so have been taken without success."

Acting as an aid or facilitator in conversation can support a person with communication difficulties to engage successfully in the decision-making process. In this role the SLT may be considered an 'interpreter' in an assessment of decision-making capacity. This can also provide a useful role model for future communication between the individual and other decision-makers (Murphy et al., 2010). It may not always be clear what, for example, 'writing key words' actually looks like in a conversation.

The SLT as implementer

An SLT may also act as an implementer following assessment, addressing areas of need or change that having been identified during the assessment process. This may include implementing dysphagia-related decisions or perhaps supporting newly-assigned Deputies in how to communicate with the person with communication difficulties (see Chapter 10)

Should a person be assessed as not having decision-making capacity for a particular decision, it is important to remember that they may still be able to express a preference. In this situation, it will be helpful for the SLT to act as an aid to communication in order for the person to express their opinions. For example, a person may clearly indicate that they wish to go home, even though it is not clear that they understand the risks or challenges associated with this. When the MDT makes a best interests decision, this wish needs strong consideration, in addition to the risks of not honouring this wish, such as: less contact with friends/family; disengagement from the wider therapeutic process; and the impact on mood and wellbeing.

A word of warning...

It is important to consider the impact of your role in the assessment of decision-making capacity and how this will sit in your current role. Morris et al. (2012) warn that, although taking on the role of assessor is a vital part of our role as SLTs, it can have a negative effect on the therapeutic relationship. Having said this, it is worth referring back to the recommendations from the MCA Code of Practice (2007). This document advocates conducting complex assessments alongside a colleague. Taking a joint approach can assist in balancing this interplay of roles and reducing the risk of a negative impact on therapeutic roles. This can also reduce bias and lend credence to assessment outcomes.

The multidisciplinary team

The following provides an idea of all those who may be part of the MDT involved in a capacity issue. It is not an exhaustive list of all those working with an individual, but does highlight those with some core responsibilities related to assessment of capacity.

Medical team

Doctors have long held a traditional role as head of the MDT, especially within the acute area of medicine. They have responsibility for the overall care of the patient and, ultimately, any medical treatments that are considered to be beneficial, thus often assessments of capacity fall to them. In addition, the MCA (2005) stipulates that the person who will be conducting a procedure should be the individual to assess the person's decision-making capacity. Since medical professionals are most frequently the person conducting a serious medical procedure, such as an operation or examination, they are often required to conduct the assessment of consent capacity themselves.

Psychiatrists

Psychiatrists may take the lead in a person's care, particularly where there is a known or suspected mental health issue. They also have a key role in assessing and managing people with dementia. They may ultimately be of the opinion that a person needs to be treated under the Mental Health Act and there are set legal procedures for this. If the person has not been detained under a 'section' then their decision-making capacity will more likely influence the management of their care. Similarly, the psychiatrist may be a key member of the team recommending that a person would benefit from an admission to hospital, thus they are frequently involved in assessments of consent capacity.

Psychologists

Psychology colleagues may conduct a range of cognitive and neuropsychological assessments. Depending on the skill-mix within a team, they may also have a role in looking at linguistic aspects of communication, particularly where an SLT is not available. This is particularly likely in psychiatric settings, including mental health of older adults, as SLTs are often not embedded in these teams. In view of their expertise and knowledge in the area of cognition, neuropsychologists are often involved the assessment of capacity itself. They may also provide a more generally supportive role where disagreements or emotional conflicts arise. They may be able to facilitate reflective discussions to help the team understand what is happening where there are differences of opinion.

Occupational therapists (OTs)

OTs may offer cognitive and perceptual assessments that add insight to a person's underlying abilities Crucially, they also see people in 'real world' settings and can assess problem-solving and safety in a number of scenarios, from using the kitchen within a ward or at home, to catching a bus. They may also look at finances with the individual. Consequently, an OT is often involved in assessments of decision-making capacity relating to finances or discharge destinations (and care needs). Where there is no psychologist within the team, the OT often has a broader remit within cognitive assessment. This demonstrates that, although professionals have different roles within the MDT, this is likely to vary across teams, depending upon their make-up and primary focus.

Social workers

Social workers have a key role in considering different living options for their clients, and working with them and the MDT to, where possible, support the choices that the patients have made. Thus, social workers may also be involved in assessments of decision-making relating to discharge destination, as well as advocating for a person in any given decision.

Solicitors

It is not uncommon for solicitors to be appointed as Deputy for individuals who do not have a family member who can take on this role. SLTs may work collaboratively with solicitors, particularly with regards to providing advice on communication needs or acting as an aid to communication.

People in the community or within acute settings may also require legal advice regarding the appointment of a lasting power of attorney, completing an advance directive or writing a will. However, it is for the solicitor to decide if they are satisfied that the person has demonstrated decision-making capacity to engage in legal matters, as stated in the MCA Code of Practice (2007):

"For a legal transaction (for example, making a will), a solicitor or legal practitioner must assess the client's capacity to instruct them. They must assess whether the client has the capacity to satisfy any relevant legal test. In cases of doubt, they should get an opinion from a doctor or other professional expert." (p. 54)

Whenever an SLT, whether working within the National Health Service (NHS) or for another type of organisation, is asked to be involved with a solicitor, either as an aid to communication or as a professional expert, it is strongly recommended that they seek advice from their manager and the organisation's legal team. Case study 1 illustrates how this type of advice can enable an effective assessment. Depending on the situation, there may be potential conflicts of interest in legal areas that the SLT is not aware of. Moreover, it could be beyond the scope of the service they are working within. Working with a solicitor is not considered a usual clinical role for an SLT, so it may be argued that the therapist should not feel pressured into doing this and only become involved if she feels competent to do so. Even as an aid to communication, the SLT's involvement could be challenged at a later date. Where the organisation decides the SLT should not be involved in a specific legal matter, a private practitioner can be sought, although this is likely to have cost implications for the individual conc+erned.

Case Study 1

Mrs E has been diagnosed with a brain tumour. She is bed bound and has severe word finding difficulties, although her receptive language is intact. She is very distressed that her will is out of date and would like to update it. The solicitor is unsure whether she has capacity and how to support her to demonstrate her decision-making capacity. There is a potentially very small window of time in which to support this individual and it has been the focus of her concern in many conversations with the MDT. After seeking advice from the legal team, it is agreed that the treating SLT can act as an 'interpreter' and that the solicitor and a medical colleague will then take a view as to whether Mrs E has been able to demonstrate capacity.

Over a series of three meetings, the solicitor felt that Mrs E had demonstrated decision-making capacity in this area, showing she understood the implications of the changes she was making, had considered other options and was consistent in her wishes across the sessions. The supportive materials used to arrive at this decision were kept by the solicitor, in case of a legal challenge. The SLT was not a witness to any of the documentation.

The benefits of working as part of an MDT in the process of assessing capacity

There is no 'right' or 'wrong' model for working as an MDT, but each situation will have an impact upon the way that team members work together. In general, working within an MDT is a complex and dynamic process. NHS England commissioned work via the National Voices campaign to find out from patients what person-centered, coordinated care within the MDT meant to them. The idea of how the team works was summarised by the campaign as "My care is planned with people who work together to understand me and my carer(s), put me in control, co-ordinate and deliver services to achieve my best outcomes" (NHS England, 2014, p. 6). Patients identified the key components required to achieving this model of coordinated care as focusing on the following topics in shared conversations:

- Goals/outcomes
- Communication
- Information
- Decision-making
- Care planning
- Transitions
- Emergencies

This work contributed to the NHS England "Multidisciplinary Team Development Guide – Working toward an effective multidisciplinary, multiagency team" (NHS England, 2014). The document was written to support services to reflect on how they practice and what sort of team they are. The guide proposes that there are four main structures to MDTs. These range along a continuum from a more unidisciplinary model where a central clinician works most directly with the patient and may call on other professionals as needed, to a transdisciplinary model where traditional roles might be broken down with acknowledged blurring of these roles to bring about the most effective care of an individual. The model and the tool that goes with this can be accessed for free via the NHS UK website at http://www.england.nhs.uk/wp-content/uploads/2015/01/mdt-dev-guid-flat-fin.pdf.

For the purposes of a specific capacity issue, a new team may need to be formed. Different models may be appropriate for different situations, and it is worth reflecting on the demands of each situation in turn using a model such as that described above. This may be the best way to identify if a person has decision-making capacity and to ensure that everything possible is done to acknowledge the capacity of an individual where it is present. Forming a new team when a person has been found not to have decision-making capacity in relation to a specific decision can ensure a more person-centered, robust decision is made in that person's best interests.

In addition to information sharing, team members may work directly together with the patient as described above in setting goals, care planning, decision-making, planning transitions and managing emergencies. As previously mentioned, the SLT may take on a number of different roles when contributing to this process in assessments of capacity: assessor, advocate, advisor and aid to communication. Joint working in this way allows for:

- A more transparent and robust assessment process, where two people have been involved in an interaction with the person being assessed. This reduces bias and increases validity.

- The opportunity to view communication and behaviours from another perspective, which can be helpful. For example, the SLT may have the view that reduced understanding is a language comprehension difficulty, while the psychologist proposes attention as a contributing factor. It could be either, or both, but trying different strategies to support the person may enable them to demonstrate capacity.

- Joint problem solving, which can contribute to a more timely outcome. Experience of more and varied situations can provide a broader view of a variety of solutions.

- Learning from one another, which can hone the skills of the team. Observing, for example, how the psychiatrist interacted with a man experiencing delusional beliefs, or how the OT examined a functional task in terms of a person's cognitive ability can allow the team to share skills and learning for the future.

By working more closely together, it is hoped that issues within the team can be dealt with swiftly and respectfully and that there will be better consensus around capacity. However, there are times when relationships within the team may become strained.

Conflict within the MDT when assessing capacity

In general, we do not examine the team dynamic unless there is a problem. There are theoretical approaches to team working and team roles that can be explored if the team wish to look in detail at how they are working together. The type of approach taken would depend upon what areas the team wishes to investigate, and depend on how static the team membership is. Some examples include The Belbin Team Roles Questionnaire (Belbin, 2010), which can be useful for an established and static team. Other more psychodynamic approaches, such as Berne's (1961) *Transactional Analysis in Psychotherapy*, or Karpman's (1968) Drama Triangle, can also be a useful way to frame thinking if there is discord within the team.

It can be useful to consider team dynamics even where the team does seem to work effectively, both to find out why it does and to check for subconscious collusion. Some questions that may be useful to ask are:

- Is there a clear team leader?

- Does this person always take the lead, or are there times when it is acknowledged someone else may be best placed?

- Does everyone feel able to share their opinions?

- Are conversations held respectfully?

- Have cliques formed, which could lead to 'block voting' or decision-making?

- Are individuals aware of their values and personal histories that may lead to bias?

It can also be useful to consider some of the key areas where conflict can arise in terms of decision-making capacity:

- Some members of the MDT find the individual to have capacity to make a specific decision, other members not.

- Poor communication between team members.

- Where a person's 'unwise' yet capacitous decision-making conflicts with the team's recommendations.

- Difference between family's view about capacity and that of the MDT.

- Disagreement within the MDT about what constitutes best interests in a given situation.

- Difference between family's view about a best interests decision and the MDT's view

Case study 2 demonstrates how poor communication across teams can result in lengthy and drawn-out decision-making, even when issues are resolved. The MCA Code of Practice (2007) makes provision for disagreements and recommends that, where possible, these are resolved quickly and internally, giving the following suggestions for achieving resolution with family members:

- Setting out the different options in a way that is easy to understand

- Inviting a colleague to talk to the family and offer a second opinion

- Offering to get independent expert advice

- Using an advocate to support and represent the person who lacks capacity, arranging a case conference or meeting to discuss matters in detail

- Listening to, acknowledging and addressing worries, and where the situation is not urgent, allowing the family time to think it over (MCA Code of Practice 2007, p. 258–9)

Case Study 2

Mr J was in hospital, following a stroke. He had severe receptive and expressive aphasia, with staff supporting him to make choices regarding basic needs, such as pictures of food to choose meals. He also had severe dysphagia and was being fed via a nasogastric (NG) tube. Two SLTs on the ward had worked closely with the medical and nursing team to see if percutaneous endoscopic gastrostomy (PEG) could be explained to him. He was unable to demonstrate that he understood what a PEG was, to show if he would be interested in having a PEG, or to show an appreciation of any risks. He was distressed by his NG tube and frustrated at times by his communication, but overall appeared to be content on the ward. His family felt that that he would want to have a PEG and that this was the way forward for Mr J, especially with a view to having him home. A best interests meeting was held with the MDT and the family, and the decision was made that PEG insertion was in Mr J's best interests and would ultimately lead to less restriction than NG tube feeding in hospital. Oral feeding was not an option at this time, as Mr J had an almost absent swallow. The procedure went ahead and discharge planning continued.

As part of the usual tests following his stroke, Mr J had a scan of his carotid arteries, which were found to be 50% occluded on the left side. He had been seen by a surgeon, who had scheduled him for surgery with a comment in the notes that Mr J had consented to the treatment. This was not discussed with the wider MDT and the stroke consultant had not been made aware of the decision. This was picked up in the MDT; it was agreed that Mr J did not have the capacity to make this decision and that the consultant, surgeon, SLT and member of Mr J's family would meet to discuss the situation further. The surgeon acknowledged that his original assessment regarding capacity had been somewhat hasty and took on board the views of the rest of the team. However, he still felt that the surgery was the best course of action. Mrs J expressed concerns about the risks and did not want her husband to have unnecessary surgery. The stroke consultant was also concerned that Mr J was on the borderline for whether this intervention was indicated (RCP Stroke Guidelines, 2012). After much discussion, a best interests decision was taken by the surgeon, stroke consultant and Mrs J, who on balance felt that the risks and benefits of the surgery were fairly even and therefore the least restrictive and least distressing option for Mr J was not to go ahead with the surgery.

Recording information

Case study 2 provides a fictional example of an unfortunately fairly common 'near miss' scenario. It demonstrates the difficulties that people with aphasia and their families may experience within the NHS, and the lack of understanding of how communication difficulties and aphasia impacts upon decision-making capacity. More generally, it highlights the need to think about how as a team we record information concerning capacity and how we share this with a wider audience. While capacity is decision-specific, there will be some areas where not being able to demonstrate capacity in one area will have an impact on other areas.

In 2010, the British Psychological Society produced a useful audit tool that breaks down the different components of making a decision with regards to mental capacity, in detail. Some services use a variation of this in its entirety to store in medical records, and this would clearly be an example of best practice. Other records of assessments of decision-making may be within the main body of the medical record, but others not recorded at all. Good practice would suggest that, as a minimum, the information should be clearly documented, in a location where others know how to find it, and which should be agreed at a local level (Table 6.1, Table 6.2).

Table 6.1 Minimum requirements for documentation of assessments of **decision-making capacity** (compiled from the British Psychological Society audit tool, 2010).

Name of assessor(s) and date(s)
What was the decision?
Who is the decision-maker?
How was the person assessed?
Were efforts made to support the person to understand the decision? Y/N
Did the person demonstrate comprehension of the information presented? Y/N
Could the person retain the information? Y/N
Could the person demonstrate an ability to weigh up the decision? Y/N
Could the person communicate the decision? Y/N
Does the person therefore have the capacity to make this decision? Y/N
If the person does not currently have capacity, is this likely to alter in the near future? Y/N

Table 6.2 Minimum requirements for documentation of **best interest decisions** (compiled from the British Psychological Society audit tool, 2010).

People involved in discussion and role
What is the decision at hand?
Has it been clearly shown that the person lacks capacity to make this decision?
Does the person have a view on what is preferable for them?
Does the family have a view on what is best (if not represented at the meeting)
What are the options?
Risks and benefits of all options
What is the least restrictive option?
Having weighed up all the above, what is felt to be the best decision?

Having a structure to the process helps to clarify people's thinking and to ensure that all the key areas are covered. However, the more complex or controversial the decision, the more information may need to be sought. Case study 3 illustrates the processes involved in appropriately assessing these types of complex issues.

Case Study 3

Mrs K had a diagnosis of dementia and a stroke that affected her comprehension. She was able to have conversations about the here and now with some strategies, e.g. keeping sentences simple and using gesture. Physically, Mrs K had a catheter and was able to sit in a chair with a pressure-relieving mattress for several hours. She could feed herself with some set-up.

She was admitted to hospital following a fall, and there were concerns that her husband may have been transferring her in a rough manner, or possibly grabbing her, as she had bruises on her arms. A safeguarding alert was raised. Mrs K was unable to provide any information about this issue and her face lit up when her husband visited. The social worker met with Mr K, who denied grabbing or hitting Mrs K, but acknowledged that sometimes he found it hard to help her out of bed. It was suggested that Mr K work with the OT on the ward to look at transfers and to see if further help was needed at home. Mr K was extremely reluctant to have a package of care. While on the ward, it was established, that for safe transfers, Mrs K needed two people to help her and therefore if she was to return home, Mr K would need more help.

Mrs K kept asking to go home and evidently missed her husband while on the ward. Her mood was beginning to decline and she was eating and drinking less and often becoming tearful. However, Mr K remained reluctant to have a package of care at home.

The SLT and the social worker worked with Mrs K over several sessions using predominantly informal assessment, to assess her decision-making capacity in regard to her discharge. She was clear she wanted to go home and that she and her husband would be 'fine', but she showed little insight into the help she was receiving on the ward and could not recall what the situation was like at home. She deferred all issues to her husband and emphasised her preference as simply wishing to go home.

It was agreed that Mrs K did not have the capacity to make the decision about her care needs on discharge. Mr K wanted to have his wife back home and was frustrated by the amount of time she had been in hospital, particularly as she seemed to be 'getting worse' and was not eating and drinking. He had worked with the OT on the ward, but had made it clear that he felt that he would be fine on his own and that the staff were being overzealous by using two people for transfers stating, "She's so tiny, I can just lift her" – attempting to demonstrate.

A best interests decision meeting was held, initially without Mr K present, given that the team needed to be able to speak frankly about their concerns.

A summary of the meeting was recorded.

People involved in discussion and roles:
Elderly Care Consultant – Dr E
GP – Dr P
Primary nurse – Bev
OT – Kate
SLT – Hannah
Social worker – Sue (main decision-maker)
Community Mental Health Nurse – John

What is the decision at hand?
Should Mrs K go home to live with her husband?
Has it been clearly shown that the person lacks capacity to make this decision? Y/N
Does the person have a view on what is preferable for them?
Mrs K would like to return home
Does the family have a view on what is best (if not represented at the meeting)?
Mr K would like his wife to return home with no extra care

What are the options?
– Mrs K to return home with no extra care

- Mrs K to return home with a package of care (4 times daily, single-handed, Mr K to be other person for transfers)
- Mrs K to return home with a package of care (4 times daily, double-handed, Mr K not to be involved in transfers)
- Mrs K to be transferred to a care home with nursing

Risks and benefits of all options.

Option 1: Mrs K to return home with no extra care

Risks:

- Mrs K continues to need 2 people to safely transfer, risk of bruising, falls and other injuries if transferred by just Mr K.
- Mr K has had relatively poor engagement with MDT, unclear if he would ask for help if needed.
- It is felt that the bruises were as a result of rough transfers, rather than elder abuse, but we are not sure of this.

Benefits:

- This is Mr and Mrs K's wish
- Fewer restrictions on timings for transfers and personal care
- What is the least restrictive option?

Option 2: Mrs K to return home with a package of care (4 times daily, single-handed, Mr K to be other person for transfers)

Risks:

- Remains unclear whether abuse occurred
- Does not help with times in between visits when Mr K may still transfer his wife alone, or when she is asking to sit out in her chair or go to bed

Benefits:

- Most closely aligns to Mr and Mrs K's wishes
- Another agency would be involved and could identify signs of Mr K not managing and any physical injuries
- Would allow for safe transfers and personal care

Option 3: *Mrs K to return home with a package of care (4 times daily, double-handed, Mr K not to be involved in transfers)*

Risks:

– Remains unclear whether abuse occurred

– Does not help with times in between visits when Mr K may still transfer his wife alone, or when she is asking to sit out in her chair or go to bed

– May be very negatively viewed by Mr K, leading to potential refusal of access/withdrawal

Benefits:

– Mrs K will be at home

– Mrs K able to get used to other carers, especially if Mr K became unwell.

Option 4: *Mrs K to be transferred to a care home with nursing*

Risks:

– Mrs K's mood will suffer – already eating and drinking less and seems depressed

– Reduced contact with husband

Benefits:

– Transfers and personal care should be carried out safely

– 24-hour care, hope would be that they could be safely responsive to personal care needs

– More supervision of Mr K, given query around physical abuse.

Least restrictive option:

Option 1 – home with Mr K and no care

Having weighed up all the above, what is felt to be the best decision?

There was much discussion in the meeting and consensus could not be reached. However, on balance, the social worker believed that Option 2 (Mrs K to return home with single-handed package of care) was the best option, taking into account:

– Mrs K's wishes

– Second least restrictive option

– *Ability to monitor for signs of rough handling/abuse.*

Points raised:

– *OT and primary nurse felt that the issue of abuse and rough handling was most important and that Mr K would not follow guidance once home. They had worked directly with Mr K over the past few weeks and had not found him to be very receptive. They were also concerned that Mr K may deny access to carers.*

– *GP had not seen previous evidence of abuse and although Mr K has strong views about his wife's care, has regularly contacted the surgery for home visits when he has had concerns, gets regular health checks, etc.*

– *SLT and Community Mental Health Nurse both felt that there would be a negative impact on Mrs K's mental and physical health should she be discharged to a nursing home. Both felt that Mrs K should be able to go home with support. However, both acknowledged caution and advocated regular monitoring.*

Further provisions also to be added:

– *Weekly social work visits for first month, frequency thereafter to be agreed*

– *Social worker and OT to meet with Mr K, to explain need for package of care and that Mrs K's ability to stay at home will depend upon this*

Case study 3 also highlights that a team may not always reach a consensus about a decision, particularly when said decisions are complex, involving significant areas of risk. In these situations, there is rarely one clear 'good' option or one clear 'bad' option. It may be more about navigating through 'various shades of grey'.

The team, in this example, is trying to anticipate future events based on the limited evidence that is available. Although there were strong feelings, the discussion was held respectfully and once a decision had been made, the team worked together to achieve the best outcome. At this time, the ultimate outcome of this type of decision remains an unknown. Yet communicating effectively as a team, and with all members of the team, is often the most important ingredient to a successful outcome. Case study 4 provides an example of how communication can easily break down.

Case Study 4

Mr P lives in a nursing home and has a brother who lives overseas. He has quite advanced dementia, but has been engaging in basic conversation, eating and drinking independently. He is mostly in bed, but sits out in the a chair for a few hours. He has what appears to be a stroke one weekend. The nursing home contact the GP. An out of hours doctor from the local GP consortium, Dr A, attends agrees that it is likely to be a stroke, but decides not to admit Mr P to hospital. Mr P now presents with severe swallowing difficulties and food and drink is running from his mouth when it is given to him. He does not appear to be able to swallow at all. His right arm is very weak and he has reduced movement in his right leg.

An urgent SLT referral is made by the nursing home, and the SLT attends the same day. Mr P is alert and asking for a drink. When offered a range of textures, he appears best able to manage a smooth yoghurt, but his swallow is very delayed. He continues to ask for a drink and so is given sips of water or tea, even though much of this is lost anteriorly. The SLT recommends to another GP, Dr B, that this gentleman is unsafe on all oral intake. He is able to engage in basic communication, but does not have capacity to make a decision about his ongoing treatment or to be aware of the risks of aspiration.

Consequently , Dr B visits and recommends to the care home that they treat him as palliative. After 2 days there is no improvement to his swallow and the nurse at the care home raises concerns about his nutrition and hydration. The staff at the care home feel that Mr P should be in hospital. They are used to caring for people with end-stage dementia, but feel that this situation is different as he has so suddenly become unable to swallow.

Another GP, Dr C, refers to a 'hospital at home service', who set up sub-cutaneous fluids. The main GP, Dr B, still feels that care is best provided at the care home, but the SLT and care home staff are becoming increasingly uneasy and are concerned that Mr P has been discriminated against and has been 'written off' due to dementia, when the main medical issue at this time is the stroke. The care home staff are worried that they are starving Mr P.

Communication between different members of the team, which so far have involved the care home, three GPs, hospital at-home team and SLT have been predominantly via telephone.

A care-of-elderly medical consultant with a special interest in stroke visited the home and assessed Mr P. By this time Mr P was significantly more frail and it was felt that on balance he should remain at the nursing home. He died peacefully a few days later.

Take a few moments to think about your reaction in this situation. Has a person with dementia received lesser treatment because of their condition? Or is the GP right to view this situation as palliative and non-reversible? What other steps should be considered?

As a result of the discord within the team, a case review was carried out, to look at what learning points there might be for future care. The following points were raised:

- Best practice is for someone with a stroke or suspected stroke to be admitted to hospital for assessment. While the original assessing GP, Dr A, had not felt that this was appropriate in this case, it was felt, on balance, that this should have been considered more as an option and that the reason not to admit was not adequately explained and documented. However, it was acknowledged that this was a difficult decision, without one clear 'best' solution.

- A consultant opinion should have been sought sooner.

- Communication via phone and notes was not always effective and a face-to-face MDT meeting to properly discuss Mr P's situation would have been preferable.

- The case had been managed in a hierarchical manner, without due consideration being given to other people's areas of expertise. This led to further fracture within the team and an irreparable sense of 'injustice'.

Conclusion

The responsibility that health professionals feel to protect people from harm can, at times, directly conflict with a person's own decision, or what is felt to be in the person's best interests. On a personal level it can be very difficult to balance respect for autonomy and protection of the vulnerable individual when assessing decision-making capacity (Lo, 1990). This is where the team can support one another emotionally and professionally. Yet working as a team raises many challenges, including differences in professional and personal opinions.

The MCA (2005) acknowledges these difficulties and provides guidance to support the management of these. As SLTs, we can be proactive in this process by reflecting not just on our own values and beliefs about a specific situation but on the role we will take within the team in a specific situation. Being transparent and maintaining clear lines of communication and documentation can go some way toward reducing the negative consequences that can arise in complex situations.

References

Belbin, R.M. (2010) *Team Roles at Work*, 2nd ed. London, Butterworth Heinemann.

Berne, E. (1961) *Transactional Analysis in Psychotherapy*. New York, Grove Press, Inc.

British Psychological Society (2010) Audit Tool for Mental Capacity Assessments. http://www.bps.org.uk/sites/default/files/documents/audit-tool-mental-capacity-assessments_0.pdf

Carling-Rowland, A., Black, S., McDonald, L. & Kagan, A. (2014) Increasing access to fair capacity evaluation for discharge decision-making for people with aphasia: A randomized controlled trial. *Aphasiology*, 28(6): 750–765.

Flew, R. & Holly, C. (2011) Has the Mental Capacity Act changed the way SLTs work? Conference Presentation at RCSLT Wales Board Professional Development Day: Best Practice in Delegation.

Jayes, M. & Palmer, R. (2013) Initial evaluation of the Consent Support Tool: A structured procedure to facilitate the inclusion and engagement of people with aphasia in the informed consent process. *International Journal of Speech-Language Pathology*. 1–10. DOI: 10.3109/17549507.2013.7959999

Karpman, S. (1968). Fairy tales and script drama analysis. *Transactional Analysis Bulletin*, 7(26): 39–43.

Lo, B. (1990) Assessing decision-making capacity. *Law, Medicine and Health Care*, 18: 193–201.

Morris, R., Jones, J., Flew, R.J. & Mackenzie, J.A. (2012). Assessing mental capacity after a stroke: One year on. Presentation at the UK Stroke Forum, December 2012

Mental Capacity Act 2005:bhttp://www.legislation.gov.uk/ukpga/2005/9/pdfs/ukpga_20050009_en.pdfThe Mental Health Act 2005

Mental Capacity Act 2005 Code of Practice (2007): http://www.legislation.gov.uk/ukpga/2005/9/pdfs/ukpgacop_20050009_en.pdf

Murphy, J., Oliver, T.M. & Cox, S. (2010) *Talking Mats and Involvement in Decision Making for People with Dementia and Family Carers: Full Report.* Joseph Rowntree Foundation. www.jrf.org.uk. Downloaded from: http://www.jrf.org.uk/sites/files/jrf/Talking-Mats-and-decision-making-full.pdf

NHS England (2014) Multidisciplinary Team Development Guide – Working toward an effective multidisciplinary, multiagency team. http://www.england.nhs.uk/wp-content/uploads/2015/01/mdt-dev-guid-flat-fin.pdf

National Voices (2013) *A Narrative for Person-centered Coordinated Care.* WEbsite viewed: https://www.england.nhs.uk/wp-content/uploads/2013/05/nv-narrative-cc.pdf

Royal College of Physicians (2012) *National Clinical Guideline for Stroke*, 4th edition. Prepared by the Intercollegiate Stroke Working Party. https://www.rcplondon.ac.uk/sites/default/files/national-clinical-guidelines-for-stroke-fourth-edition.pdf

Volkmer, A. (2013) *Assessment and Therapy for Language and Cognitive Communication Difficulties in Dementia and Other Progressive Diseases.* Guildford, J&R Press.

7 Advanced care planning:
Supporting patients to plan for their future

Anna Volkmer

Introduction

There has been increased public interest in advance care planning over recent years, perhaps associated with the increased awareness surrounding dementia. Dementia is now considered the biggest fear for people in their 50s and 60s. In the next 25 years, it is thought that around 23% of our population will be over the age of 65 and the number of people living with dementia is set to reach more than 1.4 million by 2020 (Department of Health, 2013). As cognitive impairment progresses in dementia, decision-making capacity declines and family members are increasingly required to make decisions about life-prolonging treatments on behalf of their loved one (Garand et al., 2011; Bravo et al., 2003).

Despite all this, a relatively small number of people have appointed lasting power of attorneys (LPAs), particularly for health and welfare, and even fewer have completed written advance directives (Bravo et al., 2003). The reasons for this are likely to be multifactorial, perhaps because clinicians and patients alike find it difficult to speak about these future events, or because of a lack of knowledge in general, or because of the legal complexities involved.

However, it is clear that planning for the future, such as appointing LPAs and writing advance directives, can ensure a person is able to contribute to decisions around their own lives when they no longer have the decision-making capacity to do so. Using communication aids, both high and low tech, can enable people with communication difficulties to preserve their voices and opinions at a time when their decision-making capacity may be more impaired. Research indicates that acting as an LPA and making treatment decisions constitutes a difficult and agonising choice for family members (Forbes et al., 2000; Vig et al., 2007). Thus, future planning can support decision-makers, be they health professionals deciding whether to provide a treatment or a family member who has been appointed LPA for health and welfare decisions, in making difficult decisions in the best interests of the person they are caring for.

This chapter provides an overview of advance care planning and advance directives, touching on the role of the LPA. The remainder of the chapter further discusses the role of the SLT in this area using case examples and the research literature.

What is advance care planning?

In lay terms, advance care planning is exactly what it suggests: the process whereby a person looks to the future to consider how they would like to be treated or cared for at this time (see Figure 7.1). Advance care planning is where a person who has decision-making capacity makes an advance decision to decline a specific treatment for a time when he or she no longer has capacity to make this type of decision. This includes everything from making a 'not for resuscitation' plan at the start of an admission to hospital or prior to a major surgery to writing a detailed 'advance directive' document detailing which treatments a person wishes to decline once they no longer have decision-making capacity, having perhaps been diagnosed with a progressive condition such as MS or dementia, or simply preparing for a future event.

The concept of making a written advance directive flows directly from a cultural belief in the ethical priority of self-determination (Ditto et al., 2001). But, as is usually the case in medical law, self-determination and autonomy do not always have the final word (Royal College of Physicians and British Society of Gastroenterology, 2010). This means that, in England and Wales, a person cannot legally request or demand a treatment, only decline a treatment or express a preference for a treatment.

Appointing an LPA whilst the individual still has decision-making capacity can safeguard against this lack of clarity around choosing a treatment. An LPA has authority to make decisions related to health and welfare (should it have been donated previously) when the individual cannot any longer make their own decisions. This person is able to make decisions in the person's stead, and these decisions will be respected just as a person's own decisions are respected. Should a situation arise where there is a choice of treatment options, the LPA will be able to make this choice at the relevant time, such as choosing between treatment options A and B where there is a choice, or declining treatment X should they feel this is consistent with the person's wishes and best interests.

In some ways, the idea of advance care planning is a fairly 'young' concept born in a westernised society. Moye et al. (2004) attribute this to the increase in the numbers of adults surviving to older age in these countries, and consequently the increased incidence of dementia. Advances in medical treatment and technology have resulted in people living longer and an overall ageing population. As a result of this, people are becoming increasingly concerned that a situation may arise where they may be kept alive when they would rather not be. Moye et al. also highlight that people are now wealthier yet families are living further away from one another. This can leave older adults more vulnerable to exploitation from others, both familiar peoples and strangers. Frequently, people may be most concerned about the financial affairs of their loved ones. Thus, there is increased awareness around planning for future health and welfare decisions through advance directives and LPAs.

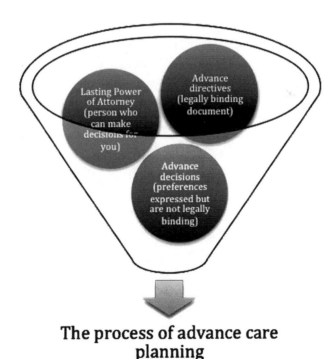

The process of advance care planning

Figure 7.1 The process of advance care planning.

The idea of these types of advance directives was first discussed in America in 1968. It was only in the 1980s that the Euthanasia Charity introduced the concept to the UK. In the UK, advanced directives were legally recognised only in 1993 in the case of Tony Bland (Airedale NHS Trust vs Bland). This case went to the House of Lords, who found that it wasn't in his best interest to stay alive. Although this case did not have anything to do with advanced directives themselves, the judge stated that courts will consider an advanced directive or statement about an individual's care when making their decision. It was not until much later that this piece of case law became legislation with the introduction of the Mental Capacity Act (MCA, 2005).

Advance decisions

What is an advance decision?

The MCA (2005) defines an advance decision as:

> "...a decision made by a person ("P"), after he has reached 18 and when he has capacity to do so, that if—
>
> • at a later time and in such circumstances as he may specify, a specified treatment is proposed to be carried out or continued by a person providing health care for him, and
>
> • at that time he lacks capacity to consent to the carrying out or continuation of the treatment,
>
> • the specified treatment is not to be carried out or continued." (Section 24, 1)

As mentioned, an advance decision cannot be made to 'have' or 'request' a treatment. An individual may express a preference for a certain treatment, such as having IV fluids at the end of life. The treating team will only consider this preference; it is not legally binding for them to follow the stated preference. In comparison the treating team is legally bound not to provide treatments that have been declined in an advance directive document.

Another valuable point to make is that advance decisions are only relevant once the individual has lost capacity, not while they are still able to make that decision themselves at the relevant and required time. The MCA (2005) attempts to address the issue of advance care planning, linking it directly to capacity and clarifying its place in health care planning and delivery.

Communicating advance decisions

Advance directives (ADs) are the written paperwork for communicating advance decisions. They are the formal and most legally-binding method of communicating these decisions. In the recent past, they have also been known as 'living wills' or an 'Advance Decision to Refuse Treatment' (ADRT). Verbal wishes expressed to a relative and then shared with the medical team at the pertinent time have little legal standing (Royal College of Physicians, 2010), although health professionals will consider what family members have advised when making best interest decisions on behalf of the patient.

Only few people have written advance directives, although many others may have recorded their wishes and beliefs on paper, video or audio-recordings in an attempt to support future decision-making. These are not legal documents but may be useful tools to gain an insight into people's past wishes and beliefs. More evidence can be sought from, for example, their religious, political and cultural background and beliefs, and their past behaviours and habits. Again, these other methods of communicating advance decisions are not legally binding but can contribute to assist decision-makers having to make a 'best interests' decision.

The Mental Capacity Act (2005) describes:

> " A decision or statement complies with this subsection only if—
>
> - it is in writing,
>
> - it is signed by P or by another person in P's presence and by P's direction,
>
> - the signature is made or acknowledged by P in the presence of a witness, and
>
> - the witness signs."

(Section 25(6). NB: "P" = person)

The Code of Practice (MCA, 2007) also suggests including details of the individual's date of birth, address, distinguishing features, GP details and a statement of when it is to be used. See the section on the SLT's role in advance care planning (p. 172) later in this chapter for more guidance on writing an advance directive.

The most straightforward approach to advanced directive documentation is to record patients' preferences around refusing specific medical treatments in specific medical scenarios. One common example might be a preference to not receive cardiopulmonary resuscitation (CPR) should a person go into cardiac arrest. Perhaps more relevant to dysphagia may be a refusal to have a nasogastric (NG) tube or percutaneous endoscopic gastrostomy (PEG) inserted should it be recommended, or refusal of antibiotics for a chest infection (Emanuel, 1991). There may even be situations where individuals decline thickened drinks or modified foods, although this is not a 'future decision' I have clinically encountered to date. Ordinarily, the decision to decline thickened fluids arises around the time of making the recommendations, as many individuals may not know of or understand this treatment before an SLT has introduced them to it.

Quite rightly, some writers have highlighted that the specificity required by an advance directive may not provide adequate guidance to decision-makers facing treatment choices that differ from those in the scenario-based directive (Brett, 1991; Reilly et al., 1994). As we may be aware, new and novel situations may arise which the person had not considered. And, indeed, making some of these life-determining decisions can be emotionally overwhelming for family members nominated as LPAs without also having to decipher what their loved one may mean in relation to a related but different decision. Many researchers instead advocate that advanced directives focus on the "general values underlying specific choices about end-of-life care" (Doukas & McCullough, 1991).

An advanced directive does not need to be made with a solicitor (an LPA does). However, it does need to be written and preferably registered with a doctor. Table 7.1 (see p. 180) highlights all the factors that make an advance directive valid. However, knowing where to start in writing an advance directive maybe more difficult. Compassion in Dying is a registered charity that has developed a form to guide a person in writing an advance directive (www.compassionindying.org.uk). This is accompanied by clear and easy-to-follow guidance notes. Four separate sections guide you through the decision-making process. Section 1 highlights several scenarios where an individual may wish to refuse treatments. Section 2 focuses specifically on pain relief and what the individual's wishes may be should they be pregnant. Section 3 provides an opportunity to comment on declining treatment related to any specific medical condition that may have already been diagnosed. And, finally, Section 4 provides the opportunity to set out an individual's values and beliefs in general terms. It also includes sections where the LPA details can be documented, and provides step-by-step guidance in completing the document, having a witness sign it, taking it to the doctor or GP and informing all the relevant people about it.

In general, an advance directive should be signed by the person making the decision. If, as is the case for many of our patients with acquired neurological conditions, they are unable to write this themselves then a solicitor can advise on wording so that someone else can sign. Many solicitors will give brief guidance on this at no cost. As health professionals it is important not to be seen to recommend a specific solicitor. Instead, it may be useful to direct people to the Law Commission website which allows you to search for registered solicitors in specialist fields. Citizens Advice and many third sector organisations, such as Speakability, can provide advice or send assistance to support people with communication difficulties in these situations. The National Health Service (NHS) website also has a lot of useful guidance in this area.

Who needs an advance directive?

"In an ideal world everyone would prepare an advance directive document specifying treatment preferences for a variety of medical conditions and end of life care" (Bourgeois & Hickey, 2009, p. 364). Yet in reality people rarely think to the future. In fact, it can be scary and confronting to do this, especially if considering one's own mortality, or a future where one is enslaved by the limitations of a life-changing illness. These are all difficult and emotive issues to consider. Often it may seem easier 'to cross that bridge when we come to it'. Indeed, Bravo et al. (2003) found it is predominantly older, white, well- educated individuals of higher socioeconomic status who do have advanced directives in place. In many other instances, people may have made informal plans or discussed their wishes with family and friends, but very few people have considered advance directives or nominating a power of attorney.

Although it would be preferable for everyone to have an advanced directive document and a nominated LPA, there are some for whom this is more pressing. Should one have been diagnosed with a life-limiting illness which may result in future potential loss of capacity or complex and risky medical interventions, this may be more necessary (MCA, 2005). In other instances, individuals with specific cultural, religious or personal preferences may wish to ensure their 'voices are heard'. This will include those who don't have a loved one who could represent them as an LPA.

How will an advance directive assist in the future?

An advance directive (AD) communicates information about a patient's values, goals, and preferences to loved ones who are faced with the challenge of making decisions on the patient's behalf. It is also important so their preferences can be communicated to health care professionals who may be faced with making serious decisions on behalf of the person who no longer has decision-making capacity. An advance directive document maintains the patient's voice in treatment decisions. It enhances the ability of 'surrogate' decision-makers to make the treatment choices that patients would make for themselves if competent, thus improving the accuracy of surrogate substituted judgement (Ditto et al., 2001).

Repeated studies have found that, without the benefit of an advance directive, both family members and physicians show substantial inaccuracy when attempting to predict patients' life-sustaining treatment preferences (Sulmassy et al., 1998). It has been found that, without having an advance directive, decision-makers are more likely to overestimate the treatment that the individual would prefer (Ditto et al., 2001). Ditto et al. highlighted that, even with advance directives, decision-makers were unable to use or interpret the information accurately to decide whether or not the individual would chose life-sustaining treatments, still often erring on the side of overestimating the care the individual would like. In short, advance directives may still fall short of fully preserving the true voice of the patient at these times but they can certainly assist in the process.

Appointing decision makers: Nominating a Lasting Power of Attorney (LPA)

The role of the LPA is described in some detail in Chapter 4, however, as a brief reminder the MCA (2005) defines this as:

> "…a power of attorney under which the donor ("P") confers on the donee (or donees) authority to make decisions about all or any of the following—
>
> • P's personal welfare or specified matters concerning P's personal welfare, and
>
> • P's property and affairs or specified matters concerning P's property and affairs,
>
> • and which includes authority to make such decisions in circumstances where P no longer has capacity" (section 9,1).

Donating a Lasting Power of Attorney (LPA) gives the designated body the authority to make decisions about the person's health and welfare when they can no longer make their own decisions. Decisions can include where they live, who visits them and the type of care they receive. If specified, it also includes making decisions about life-sustaining care (this is addressed in Section 5 of the form itself). The Office of the Public Guardian provides detailed information, including the appropriate forms (see Figure 7.2), to apply for an LPA (direct.gov.uk/mentalcapacity). Once completed, the form must be registered. It can be useful to ask a solicitor who specialises in this area of law to provide advice at this time, and a solicitor will be needed to complete this process.

In order to nominate an LPA, the individual must have the decision-making capacity to litigate for this decision. Many people with communication difficulties may need to demonstrate that they have the capacity to do so. This is where the SLT may be involved, for example in supporting an individual with communication difficulties to demonstrate that they do indeed have the decision-making skills to identify their own proxy decision-making. Chapter 10 provides a detailed discussion on how SLTs may then support and train the LPA in communicating with their loved ones.

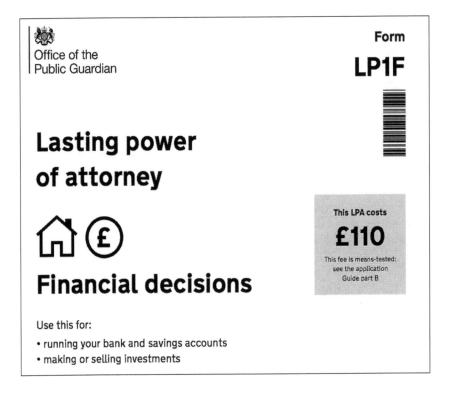

Office of the
Public Guardian

Form

LP1F

Lasting power
of attorney

Financial decisions

This LPA costs

£110

This fee is means-tested:
see the application
Guide part B

Use this for:
• running your bank and savings accounts
• making or selling investments

Figure 7.2 Sample of the first page of the lasting power of attorney (LPA) forms
issued by the Office of the Public Guardian. © Crown copyright.

The SLT's role in advance care planning

As SLTs and health professionals, our roles in advance care planning are two-
fold. We must be aware of previously-documented advanced directives, and
any nominated attorneys when making our recommendations. We are also
in a good position to provide informational counselling to patients on their
options for the future and empower them to voice their opinions about their
own future care.

When engaging in this process, it is important to understand that having
difficult conversations about the future can be emotionally challenging for
health professionals as well (Stead & McDonnell, 2015). Equally, incorporating
a refusal of treatment made prior to the SLT being involved can prove ethically

challenging. Individuals have the right to make what we may consider an unwise choice, even in relation to a future decision. On the other hand, this may make clinicians feel anxious if these decisions are contrary to the treatment recommendations being made.

As SLTs we need to recognise and consolidate these feelings in order to proceed in a professional and ethical manner. It would not be anticipated that an inexperienced clinician would take this role on without help from their colleagues and their team, through supervision and support. Even very experienced teams will continue to find themselves in challenging discussions.

The following discussion provides an outline of how the SLT may be involved with the advance decision-making process. As with the rest of this book, this is an opinion based on a collection of clinical opinions and some research literature. Others may have differing opinions on how SLT services incorporate these practices. Having a discussion with your team and coming to a consensus may be helpful.

Supporting people to make advance directives

SLTs can have an important role in empowering individuals to consider making advance directives in order to have a voice throughout the course of their care, particularly with people with progressive conditions. Advance directives could be considered both a legal document and a communication aid. Intensive care is an environment where a well-planned advance directive document could have a significant impact on patient's wellbeing and physical care (RCSLT, 2006). Poor communication between the person who is critically ill and the physician, difficulties ascertaining the person's capacity for informed consent and a failure to understand their preferences were seen to contribute to increased length of stay in intensive care and a lack of participation in end-of-life decisions (RCSLT, 2006).

Even those who have considered their own future care have rarely discussed the complex situations that may arise in these settings, and although an advance directive may not include a specific situation it could contribute to an appropriate discussion process or best interest decision. Increased communication with people about their values and preferences, particularly related to end-of-life decisions, were positively correlated with reduced length of stay (due to pro-active decisions regarding acceptance of palliative care) within the critical care environment (Dowdy et al., 1998).

Whenever possible, people with neurological disorders known to lead to cognitive impairment should be actively encouraged to consider making advance decisions (MCA, 2005) in writing, with particular reference to their preferences should cognitive function and swallowing deteriorate to the point of unsafe swallow (Jones, 2010). The MCA Code of Practice (2007) emphasises that it is for health care professionals, including SLTs, to take on the role of providing information to people who still have capacity in order to prepare them for this process. Many organisations, including the National Institute for Health and Care Excellence (NICE), also advocate this role for health professionals (including SLTs) involved in dementia care, for example. The NICE dementia guidelines (2011) state that:

> "Health and social care professionals should discuss with the person with dementia, while he or she still has capacity, and his or her carer the use of:
>
> • advance statements (which allow people to state what is to be done if they should subsequently lose the capacity to decide or to communicate) advance decisions to refuse treatment
>
> • Lasting Power of Attorney (a legal document that allows people to state in writing who they want to make certain decisions for them if they cannot make them for themselves, including decisions about personal health and welfare)
>
> • a Preferred Place of Care Plan (which allows people to record decisions about future care choices and the place where the person would like to die)." (Section 1.1.4.4)

Case study 1 provides an example of where the SLT might contribute to the advance care planning process in this way.

While it can feel uncomfortable to have these types of conversations about the future, SLTs are in a position to influence this phase of a person's quality-of-life by addressing death and end-of-life wishes. Many researchers and clinicians advocate this as a goal of therapy (Stead & McDonnell, 2015). In fact, data collected from practising SLTs working with people with semantic dementia highlight that supporting patients in this area of future planning, including decision-making in issues such as LPA, has become a routine part of speech and language therapy practice (Kindell et al.).

Case Study 1

Mr P has been referred to speech and language therapy (SLT) with a history of worsening language difficulties over the last year. His ex-wife feels his difficulties could be attributed to his alcohol consumption or his apparent anxiety. The psychiatrists feel this may be some sort of language variant of fronto-temporal dementia. He is diagnosed with logopenic variant primary progressive aphasia. Mr P explains to the SLT during the course of their therapy sessions that he now lives alone in a flat that he and his ex-wife co-own. They own a number of other properties together and have decided to maintain this financial arrangement. He has two children who live outside London and one who lives close by.

Mr P's language symptoms continue to decline over the 6 months that he is involved with the SLT. During this time he expresses some fear for the future, including how he might communicate his preferences. The SLT provides Mr P with counselling and advice on visiting his solicitor to nominate an LPA and writing an advance directive. Mr P identifies that he would like two of his children to take the role of financial power of attorney jointly. He speaks with them, and they are agreeable. He then approaches his solicitor who completes the required documentation with him. He decides not to pursue an advance directive for the time being.

Mr P is re-referred to the service 6 months later; his communication has continued to deteriorate. He is now also reporting physical symptoms, including numbness of the low limbs. The team is now concerned that he may be developing symptoms of motor neurone disease. Mr P is keen to consult with the SLT to support him in preparing for the future. He is worried about his swallowing and wishes to write an advance directive to decline any feeding tubes should they be recommended, and should he lose capacity to make such a decision. He has spoken to his medical team about this, who have voiced concerns about his current decision-making capacity given his worsening aphasia. The SLT uses a supported communication technique, employing pictures, written words and verbal discussion to assess his decision-making capacity in a joint session with the consultant psychiatrist. She photographs the pictures and written words which highlight that Mr P does have decision-making capacity to make this decision. The consultant and the SLT document the assessment in the medical notes and write a report, with the images attached. The SLT, patient and psychiatrist complete the advanced directive paperwork, placing a copy in his medical file and a copy with the patient's GP, attaching it to the report. The SLT then spends some time developing a communication passport with the patient, which includes the advanced directive paperwork and photos, all in a format that Mr P is able to use and show others in supported conversations. The communication passport includes other information over time such as information about his family and his children, who have been nominated as LPAs. Mr P and the SLT discuss how the communication passport can be developed further and revisited in the future. Although they do not add information on issues such as his preferred interests, personal history or other day-to-day choices, the SLT inserts some information on how to do this in the future.

Many SLTs advocate creating an advance directive that is also replicated in a communication book, aid or passport medium (Bourgeois & Hickey, 2009). Bourgeois et al (2009) describe using advance directives in dementia care as communication tools to assist the person with dementia in structuring communication around care plans and treatment options. They explain that external strategies such as memory and communication books support retrieval of information from long-term memory storage through the environmental triggers they provide. Memory and communication books are certainly an area that SLTs are familiar with. In this case, the therapist discusses with the patient and their loved ones what would be important to include, collecting photos and memorabilia, and developing a book of information to support memory and conversation. This may take the form of a small wallet for medical information, including an advance directive document, or family names and pictures or a detailed personal history memory book with written sentences and a picture to aid recall of particular events. This document can then support a person in conversation with other people, either as a tool the person with communication difficulties can present to convey desired details or as an aid to others to introduce a supported conversation. Bourgeois (2007) has published a manual describing the types and formats of different communication aids that can be used with people with dementia.

NOTICE OF ADVANCE DECISION CARD

1. Print this sheet out on an A4 sheet of paper or A4 card (preferable).
2. Fold along the dotted line.
3. Cut the card out from the sheet.
4. Stick together if required.
5. Fill in the card and carry it with you at all times.

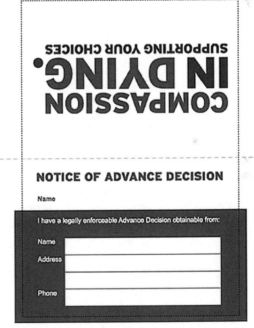

Figure 7.3 Example of a wallet card produced by Compassion in Dying (Copyright © Compassion in Dying).

There has been some research examining how people with progressive, life-limiting illness such as dementia and other progressive neurological conditions would like to express their end-of-life 'preferences' in such a passport-type document. The Royal College of General Practitioners NI who did this work found that individuals and carers rejected the concept of an 'End of Life Care Passport' as being focused on difficulties and limitations rather than on abilities and wellbeing. The group identified that the life journey with progressive illness may require a communication passport throughout, which would be updated and adapted as an ongoing process of work (Abbott, 2014; Abbott et al., 2015).

Some third sector organisations such as the Compassion in Dying charity have also developed an alert method. They provide wallet cards, which can communicate the existence of an advanced directive in more urgent situations when no one else is immediately available to do so for them (Figure 7.3). These may also be useful communication aids for people with communication difficulties.

How do SLTs respect and use an advance directive in practice?

The MCA Code of Practice (2007) emphasises that health care professionals need to be aware that a patient may have refused treatment in advance. The Code of Practice (2007) states "valid and applicable advance decisions to refuse treatment have the same legal status as decisions made by people with capacity at the time of treatment" (p. 173). For SLTs, this may mean for example that an individual with a progressive condition may have decided in advance that they would like to decline alternative feeding options such as a PEG. This in turn means that SLTs must be prepared for and endeavour to find out if such an advance decision exists, by asking family, examining medical notes or speaking to an individual's GP. If present, the advance directive document must be valid, and relevant to the proposed treatment (see Table 7.1 for guidance on what makes an advance directive valid and relevant). If this document hasn't been reviewed or updated for some time, or the person's circumstances have significantly changed, it may be useful to take more care, perhaps by consulting with anyone named on the document or someone else close to that person.

Once identified as valid and relevant, the SLT is legally obliged not to provide treatments that have been declined in the advance directive. Taking the example above, this may involve supporting the wider team to manage the least risky method of oral intake instead of a PEG. Case study 2 provides an example of how this may arise in a clinical setting.

Case Study 2

Mr C is a 56-year-old man who has been admitted to hospital and consequently intensive care following a large brain stem haemorrhage. This has left him with potentially serious long-term difficulties including dysphagia, cognitive impairment and communication impairment. The SLT involved has been assessing his swallow function and he remains unsafe for oral intake. He has had a video fluoroscopy X-ray that has confirmed these results. Mr C is given a nasogastric tube. He makes little gain in his swallow function over the next two months, remaining on sips of custard thick fluids only. The SLT suggests a long-term non-oral option such as a PEG. She feels he is unlikely to make any improvements given that he has not made any improvements in his swallow or communication. The SLT and the medical team jointly assess his decision-making capacity in relation to this issue, and in the process speak to his family who flag that Mr C's advance directive statement emphasises that he does not wish to have a PEG. It is found that Mr C lacks decision-making capacity. The team, including the dietitian, agree that in order to honour the wishes of Mr C's advance directive he will benefit from another video-fluorscopy X-ray to ascertain the safest possible oral intake. It is decided that he will be safest on small amounts of custard thickened fluids and a pureed diet, complemented by supplements to maintain his nutritional requirements. The family and the team agree this is the optimal method of honouring his advance directive statement. Mr C's nasogastric tube is removed and he remains on these recommendations.

If, however, there is any doubt as to the validity of the advance directive, then the clinician can treat the person with no risk of liability. Indeed, researchers recommend that nutritional support is never an emergency and intravenous hydration can be provided to allow time to determine the existence, validity and relevance of an advance directive (Lennard-Jones, 1999; Jones 2010). This should, however, be supported by clear documentation demonstrating that this situation has been managed in a person's best interests. It may be possible to treat a person in this way until clarity around the issue has been established. In reality, it is most likely that an SLT managing a person who has declined an NG or a PEG will be working within a multidisciplinary team.

Table 7.1 Understanding whether an advance directive is valid and relevant to the proposed treatment: Checklist.

An advance directive is valid if:	An advance directive is relevant if:
• It has not expired • As per the MCA Code of Practice (2007) it should be in writing, signed and witnessed • The person should have been over 18 years when written • The person had capacity when written • The person made the advance directive of their own accord • It is applicable to the situation at hand • It specifies which treatments are refused and in which circumstances • The person has not since contradicted this/ changed their mind. • (NB: You do not need a solicitor to make an advanced decision valid)	• The person now lacks capacity • The treatment and the circumstances around this are specified in the advance directive • There must not be reasonable grounds to believe that circumstances exist which the person did not anticipate at the time of the advance directive and which would have affected his decision had he anticipated them

(Compiled from information in the MCA, 2005 and the MCA Code of Practice, 2007)

If a health professional provides a treatment for an individual that they have specifically refused, this will be considered a form of liability in the face of a valid and applicable advance directive. This can be treated as criminal liability, tortious liability for trespass and a breach of human rights.

However, when there is doubt as to the validity or applicability of an advance directive the decision must be referred to the Court of Protection and during this period all life-sustaining treatments may be given. Doubt may arise about the individual's capacity at the time of writing the advance directive, or whether the date of the document is valid. There are examples of these in case law, such as the case of 'X Primary Care Trust v XB & YB (2012)'. In this case, a person with MND asked a health professional to support him to write an advance directive. The health professional entered an expiration date, but the judge ruled that the health professional wrote in the date without consulting the patient, thus it was deemed invalid.

An alternative to an advance directive is the appointment of an LPA for decisions related to health and welfare. This can also complement an advance directive. Should an individual wish to appoint an LPA to make significant health-related decisions, including those relating to 'life-sustaining treatment', this must be clearly stated in the lasting power of attorney document in order for it to be valid. An advance directive can take some of the more complex decisions related to 'life-sustaining treatment' in particular out of the hands of the attorney (relieving them of this difficult job). The advance directive will only be valid in this way within England and Wales if the LPA is registered first, and the advance directive is written consequently. If the advance directive is written first it will be null and void by the LPA. As SLTs, this information can be valuable, to ensure your patients are best represented and have their voice properly and legally heard.

Summary

The role of a SLT in advance care planning can be multi-faceted. Table 7.2 provides a summary of some of the roles and tasks that we should be involved in should it be required. Having provided this extensive list, guiding individuals through the initial process of developing an advance directive or appointing an LPA will mean clinicians require some knowledge about this themselves. The following brief descriptions provide an overview of the processes required in these situations.

Table 7.2 Summary of the different roles the SLT may have in the advanced care planning process.

Role of the SLT in advanced care planning
Providing information and advice including websites and written leaflets.
Counselling and advice on future decisions, which may need to be made in the course of a person's illness.
Assessment of decision-making ability to ensure someone can write an advance directive or nominate a lasting power of attorney (LPA).
Maximising the capacity of the individual to engage in advance care planning by providing communication supports (such as that described in Chapter 6).
Advocating for the rights of people with communication difficulties who have capacity throughout this process.
Supporting communication in discussions with others such as solicitors (when arranging an LPA) and medical professionals (such as the GP when an advance directive document is being discussed).
Identifying when someone has an advance directive, and considering this when making treatment recommendations.
Identifying when someone has an appointed LPA and considering this when making treatment recommendations.
Advocating for the rights of people who have made previous advance care plans, to maintain their voice and communicate their opinions in their own treatment, when they have lost the decision-making capacity to do this. This may include developing communication aids, or wallet cards such as the example shown in Figure 7.1, developed by the charity organisation Compassion in Dying.
Engaging charitable organisations such as Compassion in Dying, Speakability and others that may be able to support people in these situations.

Advance directive documents and LPAs are a legally-binding means to ensure our patients can maintain their voice in their own care. They are a way for our patients' voices to be heard and their opinions to be enforced. It is a weapon in the armoury to fight for the right for choice throughout the duration of their care.

Having said all that, many people do not have, and choose not to write, an advance directive or nominate an LPA. In these cases, the decision falls to the 'decision-maker', often the treating medical team. Yet it is always important to remember that this does not always rest on the treating team's shoulders. There are situations where a serious medical decision cannot be made by the health professionals involved, and may need to be made by a court of law.

References

Abbott, A. (2014) Communication and Continuity in Progressive, Life-limiting Illness. A Report by the Royal College of General Practitioners Northern Ireland: http://www.rcgp.org.uk/rcgp-near-you/rcgp-northern-ireland/~/media/Files/RCGP-Faculties/Northern-Ireland/RCGP-Healthcare-Communication-report.ashx

Abbott, A., Watson, M., Gingles, J., Brown, S., Brennan, J., Scott, K. & Healy, M. (2015) PA10 What i need you to know. Building a collaborative communication tool. *BMJ Supportive & Palliative Care*, 5: A22–A22.

Bourgeois, M.S. (2007) *Memory Books and Other Graphic Cuing Systems.* New York, Health Professions Press, Brookes.

Bourgeois, M.S. & Hickey, E.M. (2009) *Dementia: From Diagnosis to Management: A Functional Approach.* New York, Psychology Press.

Bravo, G., Dubois, M. & Pâquet, M. (2003) Advance directives for health care and research. *Alzheimer Disease Associated Disorders*, 17(4): 215–222

Brett, A.S. (1991) Limitations of listing specific medical interventions in advance directives. *JAMA*, 26(6): 825–828.

Compassion in Dying website (viewed September 2015) www.compassionindying.org.uk

Department of Health (2013) *Improving Care for People with Dementia.* Viewed October 2014 at: https://www.gov.uk/government/policies/improving-care-for-people- with-dementia

Ditto, P.H., Danks, J.H., Smucker, W.D., Bookwala, J., Coppola, K.M., Dresser, R., Fagerlin, A., Gready, R.M., Houts, R.M., Lockhart, L.K. & Zyzanski, S. (2001) Advance directives as acts of communication: A randomized controlled trial. *Arch Intern Med*, 161(3): 421–430. DOI:10.1001/archinte.161.3.421

Doukas, D.J. & McCullough, L.B. (1991) The values history: The evaluation of the patient's values and advance directives. *Journal of Family Practice*, 3(2): 145– 153.

Dowdy, M.D., Robertson, C. & Bander, J.A. (1998) A study of proactive ethics consultation for critically and terminally ill patients with extended lengths of stay. *Critical Care Medicine*, 26(2): 252–259.

Emanuel, L.L. (1991) The health care directive: Learning how to draft advance care documents. *J Am Geriatr Soc.* 3(91): 221–1228.

Forbes, S., Bern-Klug, M. & Gessert, G. (2000). End-of-life decision making for nursing home residents with dementia. *Journal of Nursing Scholarship*, 32(3): 251–258.

Garand, L., Dew, M.A., Lingler, J.H. & DeKosky, S.T. (2011) Incidence and predictors of advance care planning among persons with cognitive impairment. *American Journal of Geriatric Psychiatry*, 19(8), 712–720. DOI:10.1097/JGP.0b013e3181faebef

Jones, B. (2010) Ethics and artificial nutrition towards the end of life. *Clinical Medicine*, 10(6): 607–610.

Kindell, J., Sage, K., & Cruice, M. (2015) Supporting communication in semantic dementia: Clinical consensus from expert practitioners. *Quality in Aging and Older Adults*, 16(3), 153–164.

Lennard-Jones, J.E. (1999) Giving or withholding fluid and nutrients. Ethical and legal aspects. *J R Coll Physicians Lond*, 33: 39–45.

Mental Capacity Act 2005: http://www.legislation.gov.uk/ukpga/2005/9/pdfs/ukpga_20050009_en.pdfThe Mental Health Act 2005

Mental Capacity Act 2005 Code of Practice (2007): http://www.legislation.gov.uk/ukpga/2005/9/pdfs/ukpgacop_20050009_en.pdf

Moye, J., Karel, M.J.M., Azar, A.R. & Guerrera, R.J. (2004) Capacity to consent to treatment: Empirical comparison of three instruments in older adults with and without dementia. *The Gerentologist*, 44(2): 166–175.

National Collaborating Centre for Mental Health commissioned by the Social Care Institute for Excellence National Institute for Health and Clinical Excellence (revised 2011) THE NICE -SCIE GUIDELINE ON SUPPORTING PEOPLE WITH DEMENTIA AND THEIR CARERS IN HEALTH AND SOCIAL CARE, National Clinical Practice Guideline Number 42 published by The British Psychological Society and Gaskell. Downloaded from: http:// www.nice.org.uk/nicemedia/live/10998/30320/30320.pdf

Office of the Public Guardian website (viewed September 2015): www. direct.gov.uk/mentalcapacity.

Re Airedale National Health Service Trust v Bland, (1993) 1 All ER 821.

Reilly, R.B., Teasdale, T.A. & McCullough, L.B. (1994) Projecting patients' preferences for living wills: An invalid strategy for management of dementia with life-threatening illness. *J Am Geriatr Soc.* 4(2): 997–1003.

Royal College of Physicians and British Society of Gastroenterology (2010) Oral Feeding Difficulties and Dilemmas. A Guide to Practical Care, Particularly Towards the End of Life. London: Royal College of Physicians.

Royal College of Speech and Language Therapy (RCSLT) (2006) Position Paper: Speech and Language Therapy in Adult Critical Care. London, RSCLT.

Stead, A. & McDonnell, C. (2015) SIG 15. *Perspectives on Gerontology*, 20: 12–15. doi:10.1044/gero20.1.12

Sulmasy, D.P., Terry, P.B., Weisman, C.S. et al. (1998) The accuracy of substituted judgments in patients with terminal diagnoses. *Ann Intern Med*, 12(8): 621– 629.

Vig, E.K., Starks, H., Taylor, J.S., Hopley, E.K. & Fryer-Edwards, K. (2007) Surviving surrogate decision-making: What helps and hampers the experience of making medical decisions for others. *Society of General Internal Medicine*, 22: 1274–1279.

X Primary Care Trust v XB & YB [2012] EWHC 1390 (Fam)

8 Training professionals in the importance of communication to the Mental Capacity Act

Claire Devereux

> "Any assessor should have the skills and ability to communicate effectively with the person. If necessary they should get professional help to communicate with the person." (Mental Capacity Act Code of Practice, 2007, p. 54)

Introduction

This chapter starts with the premise that, as the Mental Capacity Act (MCA, 2005) applies to all professionals and carers, a basic working knowledge of this legal framework – potentially affecting any decision regarding medical treatment or care – is necessary for all. The responsibility of either demonstrating effective communication skills or seeking professional support is stipulated in the MCA Code of Practice (2007), and the role of speech and language therapy is referred to specifically where communication difficulties are present. This means that speech and language therapists (SLTs) are likely to be called on to participate in these assessments.

In practice, however, assessments of mental capacity can be done to varying degrees of quality including, in some instances, in a rather superficial way. But to undertake these assessments, in a way that meets not just the requirements of the MCA Code of Practice (2007) but the 'spirit' of the MCA (2005), requires skilled interaction. Where there is the presence of communication impairment then this interaction requires even more consideration – and competence. It can be easy to state that some people lack the capacity to make a decision. More to the purpose, perhaps, is to ask what it means to take all practicable steps to support the person being assessed, before a judgement is made.

Why is communication important in relation to the MCA (2005)?

The House of Lords post-legislative scrutiny report (2014) stated that the MCA (2005) was "a visionary piece of legislation for its time, which marked a turning point in the statutory rights of people who may lack capacity" (p. 6). Placing the individual at the heart of the decision-making process, by presuming capacity unless proven otherwise, and supporting the individual to make decisions for themselves as far as possible "signified a step change in the legal rights afforded to those who may lack capacity, with the potential to transform the lives of many" (House of Lords, 2014, p. 6). This was further enhanced by recognising that people with impairments were entitled to take risks and make poor decisions 'like others', and that unwise decisions were not to be used as indicators of a lack of capacity. The conferring of these rights is 'the empowering ethos' of the Act.

In terms of practice and implementation, however, there is an extensive need for improvement. The need for overall improvement in implementation was emphasised by House of Lords Scrutiny Committee Chairman Lord Hardie (2014) who stated: "The committee believe that the [Mental Capacity] Act is good and needs to be implemented. What we want to see is a change in attitudes and practice across the health and social care sector which reflects [its] empowering ethos" (http://www.parliament.uk/business/committees/ committees-a-z/lords-select/mental-capacity-act-2005/news/mca-press- release---13-march-2014/).

This House of Lords post-legislative scrutiny report concluded that, whilst the MCA "embodies the intention to embed in the law the principal that everyone has the right to make their own decisions" (p. 33) the implementation of this principal was 'patchy'. Part of this 'patchiness' was in the variable quality of the assessments, with communication expertise identified as a factor. The – not terribly surprising – conclusion was that: "…the best capacity assessments are by people (who know P and) who have experience and training in communicating with people with disabilities" (p. 38).

Where decision-making capacity assessment and communication impairment meet, the literature reflects the lack of knowledge around communication barriers in our fellow health professionals. In their study of hospital doctors' rationales for inclusion or exclusion of patients in their own resuscitation decision (i.e. when considering if they should or should not be resuscitated), Hurst et al. (2013) reported a finding they described as 'of concern', namely, the invoking of communication barriers "even when based on language or an absent dental prosthesis" as a reason for not including patients in these decisions.

A consistent finding from the Mental Health Foundation (2012) in their review of mental capacity literature was the recommendation that social and health care staff and independent mental capacity advocates (IMCAs) should receive specific training in communication skills. Indeed, Carling-Rowland et al. (2014) demonstrate the positive impact that such training can have in their study where mental capacity assessors who did receive training in communicating with people with aphasia were found to more accurately assess an aphasic person's decision-making capacity. However, in general, the training that staff receive in how to use the Mental Capacity Act is inconsistent and non-standardised across different settings (McVey, 2014).

As a profession, we need to share examples of the type of research Carling-Rowland et al. (2014) describe as well as examples of good clinical practice. Our aim must be to move practice closer to embodying that 'empowering ethos' of the MCA (2005), and one of the ways to do this would be by training health and social care colleagues in how best to communicate with people with communication impairments.

In other words, training for people who are going to be interacting with people with communication difficulties, trying to address complex and dynamic needs and situations, will go some way to improving the quality of mental capacity assessments. This could in turn improve the protection of the right to autonomy of people with communication impairments. It could also support people to better participate in the decision-making process when and if they lack capacity to make that autonomous decision. SLTs could provide this training in communication, as well as directly supporting and working with individuals who are being assessed.

At the same time, we as clinicians may need support and training ourselves, in order to develop our knowledge and skills in this area. There is not a lot of literature regarding training for SLTs in the area of capacity assessment, and what there is suggests current gaps: in knowledge, available guidelines and published tools, as well as variable levels of confidence amongst clinicians (Ferguson et al., 2010). Carling-Rowland and Wahl (2010) advocate that SLTs should be at the forefront of capacity evaluation and practice. They highlight a need for training and education for SLTs themselves, to enable them to incorporate this work confidently into clinical practice.

This chapter therefore attempts to provide a framework for thinking about the skills and knowledge necessary for SLTs to feel they can develop competencies and guidelines in this area of work, as well as looking at how the profession can contribute to development and training for other professions.

SLTs and the Mental Capacity Act: Where are we in SLT? (Or, how capable do *you* feel?)

An anecdote to start with: when I asked an Adult Social Care colleague their opinion on obtaining SLT involvement in mental capacity assessment, their response was: "Well, it might be helpful, for a start, if the speech therapist didn't run a mile." One professional, one time, one remark, sure, and I do not think this reflects general practice. But I do wonder if it might reflect an impression of an anxiety about this work, and I feel it could be helpful to recognise that *some* therapists may feel hesitant about participating in the process of mental capacity assessment. In fact, a lack of education and expertise in the legal process was cited by SLTs in a study (Carling-Rowland & Wahl, 2010) as a reason for hesitancy and even reluctance to participate in assessments of mental capacity for people with acquired communication disorders. Looking at possible reasons can highlight areas for learning and skill development. Mental capacity assessment is considered a legal process, not a psychological evaluation or a therapeutic intervention. However, in practice the assessment of capacity is often a clinical process (Herbert, 2010). This can set up a tension for the therapist in working with these patients: are we undertaking a legal process – or therapy? Or both? Another cause of the 'fear' might be the responsibility inferred by the recognition of working within this legal framework, summed up succinctly in the question, "What if you got it wrong?" (Ferguson et al., 2010). Feeling uncertain as to whether an SLT should be involved in the assessment process, when this should happen, and how far this should extend, can also contribute to this overall anxiety. These concerns are reflected in the study by Carling-Rowland and Wahl (2010) where SLTs reported they were not sure of their own eligibility to carry out evaluations of mental capacity with communication-impaired clients.

Participation in capacity assessments requires a clinician to take responsibility and meet certain expectations, as in any other clinical intervention undertaken. There is some evidence in the literature to support an awareness of gaps in knowledge and understanding about capacity assessment among health professionals in general (Morris et al., 2012). Variations in experience and confidence and competence as well as specific theoretical knowledge of working within the MCA framework are likely to impact on how professionals approach capacity assessment – for example the difficulty of balancing 'enablement' with 'protection' – which can result in compromising the aim of supporting an individual's autonomy (McVey, 2014). Compare this position with our social work colleagues. My own clinical experience is that they have been able to give me clear, well-defined guidance regarding the legal processes about mental capacity and decision-making (when I haven't been running away from them, that is). Social workers can be a great source of information, as can the assigned MCA lead or representative in your trust.

(Thinking about) 'Decision-making' v. 'capacity'

However comfortable we as SLTs feel about the task of 'assessing an individual's capacity', it is now a recognised reason for referral to speech and language therapy (Royal College of Speech and Language Therapists, 2014). It has been suggested in an earlier chapter that assessing people's capacity to make decisions is part of what we do as therapists every day. Perhaps it can be useful to re-frame what we are being asked to do by participating in capacity assessment. That is, to see our intervention primarily as being with a patient who is required to try and make and communicate a decision. This may sit more naturally within an SLT's practice, in terms of the role we see ourselves having in supporting and facilitating (as opposed to purely 'testing/examining'). Does supporting someone to make a decision if they are able to do so by giving them every communication support and facilitation that they require sound more like our 'everyday' business? From my own practice, I'd venture: "Yes." Chapter 6 considers the breadth of our role in capacity assessments in more detail.

Thinking about training

Evidence from both published and clinical practice suggests that SLTs may be required to contribute to or participate in assessment in different ways, depending on the specific situation and the specific decision to be made. This can lead to a range of roles and demands on the therapist (Ferguson et al., 2010) from interpreter to assessor to advocate, to name a few, for an array of decisions to do with health, finance and social care. Some of these roles and areas may be very familiar to therapists and others may pose a challenge. The following sections will attempt look at and address possible learning points for therapists new to this area of work.

The SLTs role in mental capacity assessment

As highlighted in Chapter 6, the SLT may take on a number of different roles in the assessment of decision-making process including: advocate, assessor, advisor, educator, or interpreter amongst others (Ferguson et al., 2010). The decision in question may be wide ranging and outside the remit of routine speech and language practice; it could be about, e.g. medical treatments (outside SLT interventions), finances, safety issues, legal proceedings, accommodation or placement destinations, family conflict or issues, other processes such as safeguarding adults. This is not necessarily so relevant to our learning. We can use the 'role' we have been asked to fulfill as a guide when considering our learning needs. Case studies 1 and 2 illustrate these different learning needs for different clinical scenarios. Table 8.1 provides further guidance for SLTs working in the area of capacity assessment.

Case Study 1

Mrs A needs to make a decision; Mrs A has aphasia. She is in hospital. Her surgical team says she requires a surgical procedure. They have been unable to ascertain whether she is able to give consent. The SLT is asked to assess Mrs A and evaluate her communication in order to provide support for Mrs A and the surgical team member to have a conversation to see if she can participate in a decision about surgery. In order to provide this information, the SLT needs to identify communication needs and identify appropriate support and strategies – this may entail undertaking assessment of Mrs A's communication. This is a core skill for an SLT. In addition, the SLT may benefit from a basic understanding of the MCA (2005) test for capacity, i.e. that Mrs A needs to understand information about the decision whether or not to have surgery, to retain that information long enough to be able to make the decision, to weigh up the information and to communicate the decision. The SLT's role here could be seen as educator and advisor for medical colleagues.

Case Study 2

Mr B has dementia. He is currently under section on an acute mental health ward. His treatment will be coming to an end and the team plans to transfer him to residential care with a Deprivation of Liberty Safeguards (DoLS) authorisation should he lack decision-making capacity. He has expressed a wish to go home. His mental health team and social worker request the SLT to complete an assessment of his decision-making capacity jointly with them, as it is unclear whether he understood the questions put to him when the capacity assessment was initially attempted. The social worker is aware that communication support is indicated to ensure that all practicable steps are taken to support Mr B to see if he can make this decision. If he cannot, the team will support him to participate in a decision in his best interest. The roles here may range from educator and advisor, to interpreter, assessor and advocate. The SLT will require knowledge of the text for capacity, and will benefit from an understanding of the process of best interest decision-making and DoLS as described in the Mental Capacity Act (2005) and any updated legislation since then.

Knowledge and competencies

The British Psychological Society & Social Care Institute for Excellence Audit Tool for Mental Capacity Assessment (2010) emphasises the following competencies which would be expected of anyone carrying out an assessment of mental capacity:

- Have a good knowledge base and working understanding of mental capacity, the Mental Capacity Act (2005) and of the requirements of the particular decision-making situation
- Have undertaken any mandatory training and have the specific knowledge and skills required for each of the instruments they use
- Be aware of any limitations that may affect the reliability, validity and generalisability of the assessment when not using formal assessment tools, e.g. if conducting interviews or using observational data; and
- Receive supervision.

Table 8.1 Key learning points for participation in decision-making capacity assessment and support.

Issue of concern	Key learning points
Assessment of decision-making capacity	Knowledge of the 2-stage test outlined in the MCA (2005); (see Chapters 2, 4 and 5 for a detailed review)
Advance decision-making, particularly for nutrition and hydration issues	Understanding of advance decisions and advanced directives in the MCA (2005); (see Chapter 7)
Restricting someone from doing something, eating something or going somewhere	Knowledge of current updates on Deprivation of Liberty Safeguards (DOLS) legislation, which at the time of writing is currently under review (see Chapter 3, or consult with your MCA-DOLS representative at work)
Making a decision when someone doesn't have decision-making capacity	Best Interests Decision Processes outlined in the MCA 2005 (see Chapter 3). Awareness of how this relates to LPA and Deputy roles
Who can legally make medical and or financial decisions if the person no longer has decision-making capacity	Awareness of the role and responsibilities conferred by holding an LPA or Deputy role (see Chapter 3, and how SLTs can support them in Chapter 9)
Who can represent a person who lacks capacity and has no family or friends to support them	Knowledge of the role of the Independent Mental Capacity Advocate (IMCA) (see Chapter 3, and later in this chapter for advice on how the SLT may support an IMCA)
What about really big decisions such as withdrawing and withholding life-sustaining nutrition and hydration	Knowledge of the role of the Court of Protection (see Chapter 3)

When you say it like that...

For SLT professionals, perhaps the first step is to recognise where we have knowledge and skills and what other knowledge and skills are needed for working in this area. An argument has been made earlier in this book that asking or checking for consent for our own intervention with a patient with communication impairment is something intrinsic to our approach as SLTs.

We use our specialist knowledge of communication to adapt how an individual patient needs information presented and we can judge whether they have understood. We continue to facilitate, interpret and check this throughout our interaction with them. This fits neatly within the framework of the MCA and the assessment itself.

Training co-workers, colleagues and other assessors

It is recognised that most capacity assessments are carried out by professionals other than SLTs, even when a person may have communication difficulties. Thus those who do carry out the assessments may benefit from training in communication skills (Carling-Rowland et al., 2014). Yet compared with conversation partner training for aphasia, for example, there is not much reported about provision of training for assessors of mental capacity. This seems understandable given how recently the MCA (2005) was brought into legislation. The following section looks at the provision of training by SLTs. I will demonstrate how the profession's specialist knowledge and skills add 'value', with an example of an introductory training session for social work practitioners.

How SLTs add value

The value of specific communication-based training is illustrated in a study by Carling-Rowland et al. (2014) where social work assessors of mental capacity were trained in facilitative and supportive communication techniques. Training included developing skills in acknowledging and revealing capacity by enabling the person with aphasia to understand and communicate. The social workers were then asked to assess the capacity of a person with aphasia to make a specific decision on their placement, as were a second group of social work assessors who did not receive the training (all the people with aphasia had had their capacity on this question already established – i.e. they had capacity to make this decision). The first group used adapted information and facilitation techniques that they had been trained in, which resulted in increased accuracy in the assessment of an aphasic person as having capacity when compared to the second, untrained group. The significant difference in predicting whether capacity was determined appeared to be whether the assessor had received the training (or not) rather than the severity of language deficit or how experienced the assessor was. A salient finding was that a relatively young (42-year-old) competent adult was found to lack decision-making capacity by most of the untrained assessors. This emphasised that the communication barrier existed on the side of the untrained assessor rather than the person with aphasia. It also highlighted the significance of this type of training; the authors felt that should this lady have been found to lack decision-making capacity in a clinical setting there would have been a very real risk that she would have been placed in a care facility. In addition to this specific example on training there is evidence in the research literature that, if information is presented in 'adapted for access' formats, this can help people in understanding information regarding their healthcare (Rose et al., 2012). These findings support the argument for specialist provision of training for assessors in communication techniques

Language: "It's Complicated"

The complexities of language are widely recognised, particularly in the area of research. Pinker (1995) describes language as "a system of extraordinary complexity". Kraat (1987) underlines this with "the recognition that communication through non-conventional means is a complex process that requires more than the provision of a technical aid or device" (p. 5). Therefore, it is reasonable to expect that supporting someone with a problem in this 'extraordinarily complex task' is going to require a specialist and skilled approach.

Without the specialist knowledge of how speech and language and communication work, one can make false assumptions that lead to the wrong conclusions. Indeed, I have experienced examples of this in clinical practice where confusion about speech and language processes made by medical professionals led to misunderstandings or misconceptions. For example, during a demonstration of an artificial larynx the junior doctor asked, "How does it know which words to say?" On another occasion, when discussing a patient who had severe expressive and receptive aphasia secondary to a brain tumour and who was unable to generate written or spoken words, the SLT was asked "but can't you give her a machine to talk for her?"

We may assume other professionals know more about communication than we think; it is not uncommon to be asked to explain the difference between speech and language, something we may consider common knowledge. Indeed, during a recent conversation about a patient where assessment indicated the patient was having difficulties with different grammatical language structures, the community mental health nurse stated, "I've never thought of language in terms of different parts/structures – I thought 'not' would be easy!"

What training might assessors find most helpful?

'All practicable steps'

There are significant preconceptions and misconceptions about the ability or inability of an aphasic person to make their own decisions. Yet it is unlikely that a person who is deaf or unable to speak the language of the country they are being treated in would be viewed in the same way (Parr et al., 1997). Although these communication barriers are quite different they also have similarities, and introducing SLTs as the translators or interpreters may remove some of the assumptions around incapacity associated with communication difficulties.

According to the MCA (2005), information is to be provided in a way that is appropriate to the person's circumstances, e.g. using simple or modified language, visual aids or other means. Thinking about what people might need in terms of training, the following section highlights that it is not enough only to describe adaptations to the presentation of information. Without a basic underlying knowledge of how communication works, these adaptations may be inappropriately applied and therefore ineffective (recall the example above of the basic lack of understanding: "Why can't a machine talk for someone?"). In a recent example from a regional training session for best interest assessors, the session began with looking at what communication is, in terms of message and information exchange (Devereux, 2015, unpublished). This promoted the idea that having an appreciation about how communication usually works will support an understanding of the different ways it can go wrong and, consequently, the specific approaches that might help. Two case examples – persons 'A' and 'B' –were introduced and explored in detail throughout the session. The aim was to give a foundation for some understanding into the complexity of communication whilst grounding it from the start in a clinical context.

The following slides are given as examples with which to start explaining this complex process. One of the aims is to try and give people the experience of thinking about language in a 'conscious' or 'extrinsic' way.

What do we mean by communication?

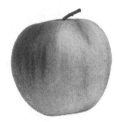

Starting with the idea of communication as one idea passed to another

Ideas – images created from memories and experience as we go through life

'apple' = 'concept' memory   *fruit, green, pie*   *(possibly computer?)*

'apple' = 'episodic memory   *'I ate one an hour ago'*

Ideas can be though of as a collection of nonverbal images

- I like apples
- I'd like one now
- To get an apple, I need to pass this idea **'apple'** on to someone else...

And consider 'what someone needs to communicate an idea' and 'what someone needs to understand an idea'.

To express:

- Form the idea
- Find word(s) that match the idea in the language area in the brain
- Brain instructs movement in muscles in mouth, throat and chest to produce the words: 'I would like an apple'

To understand:

- Need to be able to hear
- Sounds heard are sent to language area match against memory for words
- These matches are translated into images in listener's mind and they now understand the idea

Equally, the training attempted to illustrate how individuals may seem capacitous yet actually not have the skills required in the MCA assessment of understanding, recall, weighing up and communication. One small experiment is to ask someone to read a nonsense sentence aloud. This illustrates how people may seem to understand when they can 'say the words', yet actually do not understand the meaning.

> Jag hoppas att dina stolar är bekväma

This means 'I hope that your chairs are comfortable' (chosen as, phonemically, it is quite easy to read aloud for an English-speaking audience). The exercise gives trainees an 'experience' of reading aloud without any meaning and therefore is an example of how communication is driven by different distinct processes, e.g. speech without understanding!

Case examples

Using the above concepts of 'what someone needs to communicate an idea' and 'what someone needs to understand an idea', participants were encouraged to consider the case examples of Person A and Person B. The participants were encouraged to 'map' A and B's communication skills and impairments using this simple needs-based framework.

Case example Mr A

- Mr A
- 60 years old
- Logopenic aphasia (sub-type Alzheimer's disease)
- Expressive and receptive dysphasia
- Safeguarding involving family, finances, alleged abuse and living situation

SLT requested by treating team to assess capacity to:

1. Participate in safeguarding process
2. Express any choice about his finances
3. Express choice about residence
4. Express any choice about who he does and does not want to be involved in both of the above processes

---

SLT assessment

- To identify the levels of impairment and ability to identify approach that would be likely to be the most supportive and facilitative

Results:

- Good 'social' communicator. Able to use voice, and words when they are said are clear and intelligible, but severe word-finding difficulties. Can name some pictures but, e.g. a radio = 'um.. it's not for TV. Yes/no unreliable - better with nonverbal support, e.g. pictures. Unable to write.
- Understanding: Simple sentences and words with picture support and visual prompts. Assessment and other clinicians reported difficulty with following verbal instructions only. Carer gave example of gestural prompts needed when washing and undressing.

How does Mr A do?

To express

- Form the idea
- Find the word(s) that match the idea in the language area in the brain
- Brain instructs movement in muscles in mouth, throat and chest to produce the words: 'I would like an apple'.

To understand:

- Needs to be able to hear
- Sounds heard are sent to language area matched against memory for words
- These matches are translated into images in listener's mind and they now understand the idea

Strengths, abilities

Good understanding of pictures
Hearing OK
Sight OK
Can articulate words clearly
Can name/generate some words when shown pictures
Facilitated by clear gesture
v

Impairments/disabilities

Difficulty understanding spoken words, instructions
Very poor at generating words without pictures or other prompts

Communication aids for this case example were also discussed and a Talking Mat © was introduced, with an explanation and demonstration (see Figure 8.1 for an example of a Talking Mats© tool in action).

This example looked at a decision of complexity required of a person with significant expressive and receptive language impairment. Showing how using Talking Mats© elicited communication that gave a clear indication of A's feelings and preference, illustrated an 'unmasking' of competency by using adapted communication techniques. Key points were emphasised, such as careful planning of resources and assessment being carried out by two practitioners so that responses are accurately recorded. The issue of reliability in using the Talking Mats© was raised by the trainees, and addressed with reference to the literature on the use of Talking Mats© and suggestions of using the tool repeatedly (Murphy et al., 2007).

Person 'B' was then presented, using a 'basic template' for communication skills, with participants again being asked to 'map' the person's abilities and skills.

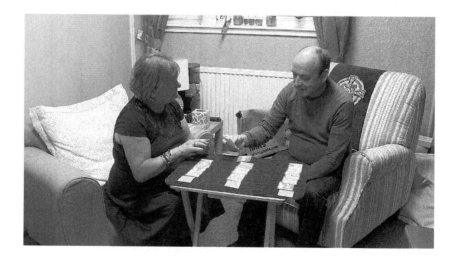

Figure 8.1 Example of how Talking Mats© can be used to support people in expressing their decisions (reproduced by permission of J. Murphy, www.talkingmats.com).

Case example Ms B

- 72 years
- History of stroke
- Severe dysarthria, dysphonia, dysphagia, saliva management problems (severe), usies litewriter and letter chart to spell out words and sentences and converse with others. Some head nod/shake and hand gesture for yes/no but requires confirmation by other means. Able to point but not always clearly due to limb weakness.
- Due to difficulties with eating, swallowing and managing saliva, Ms B wants to eat privately with no-one present in her room
- Wants to eat toast and biscuits and other foods presenting a choking risk
- Risks when not 'allowed' these, e.g. refusing personal care
- Ms B also wishes to return to her own home
- Ms B's capacity to make these decisions were addressed separately by different practitioners, with SLT participation and consultation

How does Ms B do?

To express:
- Form the idea
- Find the word(s) that match the idea in the language area in the brain
- Brain instructs movement in muscles in mouth, throat and chest to produce the words: 'I would like an apple'

To understand:
- Needs to be able to hear
- Sounds heard are sent to language area match against memory for words
- These matches are translated into images in listener's mind and they now understand the idea

Strengths, abilities

Good understanding of spoken words and sentences
AAC user - able to type words/sentences
Litewriter with voice output
Hearing? some difficulty reported
  versus

Impairments/disabilities

Very poor articulation - unable to speak words
Gestures are difficult to understand due to limb weakness
Positioning impacts upon positioning of hands for operating Litewriter

Fatigue affects hand and finger control, speech and accuracy reduced
Unable to express an understanding of risk to own person or own health in previous
discussions, suggesting reduced insight

Assessment
Carried out with social worker

Asked structured questions to assess whether Ms B demonstrated understanding of the risks
and the consequences of the risks
Ms B engaged fully with the assessment
Ms B typed her responses in full, also used some hand gesture and head nod/shake

Result

Ms B was able to respond to all questions using her Litewriter
Ms B was unable to demonstrate understanding of risks or consequences
Ms B's responses indicated a lack of insight into the risks identified with the decision

Ms B:	Let me have toast
SLT:	Do you know why I recommend you do not have toast?
Ms B:	Paranoia?
SLT:	I advised you don't have toast because of your dysphagia and because you eat alone and you are at risk of choking on toast
Ms B:	No. It's paranoia.
SLT:	If you had someone with you when you were having a meal that would help reduce the risk of you choking with no-one to help you. How about a member of staff sitting outside your door with it open a little?
Ms B:	It takes up staff time – [for them] to sit outside, better they pop in – [from] time to time
SLT:	Do you think you are at risk from choking?
Ms B:	It is non-life threatening choking
SLT:	Choking can be a threat or risk to your life
Ms B:	This is non-life threatening choking only

This example shows person B's (in)ability to weigh up the information due to her lack of insight, and although she performed well otherwise she was deemed to lack capacity.

The above examples were used to introduce the idea of the complexity of language and communication and different types of facilitation and support. A subtle – or perhaps not-so-subtle – point was that severity of linguistic impairment does not always correlate with capacity.

Conclusion

Recognising how a person communicates and their particular conversational conventions is key for any successful interaction. Misunderstandings and misinterpretations can significantly disadvantage a more vulnerable conversation partner (Kraat, 1987). A stark example of this, described by Scollon and Scollon (1980, cited by Kraat, 1987), illustrates the significant impact that this can have. They describe an interaction between English businessmen and representatives of the First Nation Athabaskan people. Both spoke English but used different pause time patterns in conversation, with the English using a shorter pause time and the Athabaskan speaker waiting for a longer pause. The English speaker waited for a second or less before speaking, the Athabaskan speaker waited for a longer period and missed their turn. The Athabaskan speaker also used a longer pause mid-utterance, which was interpreted by the English speaker as a signal to take their turn again. By only being allowed little more than a brief statement before 'losing the floor' the Athabaskans were at risk of being viewed as having 'no ideas of their own to communicate' (Pauwels, 1995). Clearly the misinterpretation resulted in an inequitable interaction: the Athabaskan speakers had less conversational 'turns' and therefore less opportunity to convey their message. One can imagine the impact this would have had on the lives of this people. Interrupted, not allowed a turn, and viewed as not having one's own ideas to express... a scenario only too familiar to people living with communication impairment.

This chapter started with the premise that SLTs – in fact, all health care professionals – need to be aware of and understand the mental capacity assessment process and framework. There is also a growing awareness of the specialist skills that SLTs can bring to this process, to support both the person and colleagues and other professionals. What is unarguable is that it is a process which is dependent, to a significant degree, on the communication skills of both assessor and assessed.

There will be ongoing challenges faced by assessors of all disciplines, including issues such as time restrictions and bed pressures. It is not uncommon for a person to question the time spent on using tools such as communication aids and make requests such as 'is there an alternative method the SLT can suggest? The assessment is taking hours!' It is our role as SLTs to continue to advocate for the needs of our patients and emphasise the value and competence of many of our patients. It is a patient's right to make a choice, if they are able (MCA, 2005). Training other disciplines in the art of communication is part of breaking down these barriers.

References

British Psychological Society and Social Care Institute for Excellence (2010) *An Audit Tool for Mental Capacity Assessment.* London, The British Psychological Society.

Carling-Rowland, A., Black, S., McDonald, L. & Kagan, A. (2014) Increasing access to fair capacity evaluation for discharge decision-making for people with aphasia: A randomised control trial. *Aphasiology*, 28(6): 750–765.

Carling-Rowland, A. & Wahl, J. (2010) The evaluation of capacity to make admission decisions: Is it a fair process for individuals with language barriers? *Medical Law International*, 10(171); 171–190.

Devereux, C. (2015, unpublished) Communication and capacity assessment. Presentation at South-East Region Best Interest Assessor Forum, May 2015.

Ferguson, A., Duffield, G. & Worrall, L. (2010) Legal decision-making by people with aphasia: Critical incidents for speech pathologists. *International Journal of Language and Communication Disorders*, 45(2): 244–268.

Herbert, C. (2010) Consent and capacity in civil cases. In Jennifer M. Brown & Elizabeth A. Campbell (Eds) *The Cambridge Handbook of Forensic Psychology.* Cambridge: Cambridge University Press.

House of Lords (2014) Select Committee on the Mental Capacity Act (2005). Report of Session 2013–2014. Mental Capacity Act 2005: Post legislative scrutiny. Published by the Authority of the House of Lords. London, The Stationery Office.

House of Lords Scrutiny Committee Chairman Lord Hardie (2014) Press release statement viewed online September 2015 at: http://www.parliament.uk/business/committees/committees-a-z/lords-select/mental-capacity-act-2005/news/mca-press-release---13-march-2014/

Hurst, S.A., Becerra, M., Perrier, A., Perron, N.J., Cochet, S. & Elger, B. (2013) Including patients in resuscitation decisions in Switzerland: From doing more to doing better. *Journal of Medical Ethics*, 39(3): 158–65.

Kraat, A.W. (1987) *Communication Interaction Between Aided and Natural Speakers: A state of the art report.* Trace Research and Development Centre University of Wisconsin Madison.

McVey, J. (2014) Written evidence to Mental Capacity Act Select Committee. Written Evidence Vol 2, 1072-1076, House of Lords. London, The Stationery Office.

Mental Capacity Act (2005) http://www.legislation.gov.uk/ukpga/2005/9/pdfs/ukpga_20050009_en.pdfThe Mental Health Act 2005

Mental Capacity Act 2005 Code of Practice (2007) http://www.legislation.gov.uk/ukpga/2005/9/pdfs/ukpgacop_20050009_en.pdf

Morris, R., Jones, J., Flew, R.J. & Mackenzie, J.A. (2012) Assessing mental capacity after a stroke: One year on. Presentation at the UK Stroke Forum, December 2012.

Murphy, J., Gray, C.M. & Cox, S. (2007) Talking Mats: The effectiveness of a low technology communication framework to help people with dementia express their views. *Journal of Assistive Technologies*, 1(2): 30–34.

Parr, S., Byng, S. & Pound, C. (1997) *Talking about Aphasia: Living with loss of language after stroke.* Milton Keynes, Open University Press.

Pauwels, A. (1995) *Cross-cultural Communication in the Health Sciences: Communicating with migrant patients.* Australia, Macmillan Education.

Pinker, S. (1995) Language acquisition. In L.R. Gleitman & D.N. Osherson (Eds) *An Invitation to Cognitive Science: Language.* Cambridge, Massachusetts: MIT Press.

Rose, T., Worrall, L. & McKenna, K. (2003) The effectiveness of aphasia-friendly principles for printed health education materials for people with aphasia following stroke. *Aphasiology*, 17(10): 947–963.

Royal College of Speech and Language Therapy (2014) Submission from the Royal College of Speech and Language Therapists to the Department of Health, Social Services and Public Safety and the Department of Justice's Consultation on proposals for the Draft Mental Capacity Bill, Northern Ireland. http://www.rcslt.org/governments/docs/draft_mentalcapacity_bill

Talking Mats information and resources: http://www.talkingmats.com/

The Mental Health Foundation (2012) *Mental Capacity and The Mental Capacity Act 2005: A Literature Review.* London, The Mental Health Foundation.

9 Information, advice and training:
Supporting carers and family members in engaging in the processes around the Mental Capacity Act and their new future roles

Anna Volkmer

Introduction

> "People and their right to make decisions are at the center
> of the MCA." (Graham & Cowley, 2015, p. 33)

Putting people at the centre of the Mental Capacity Act (MCA, 2005) includes considering the needs of carers, family and loved ones around the person involved. Often these people will hold the key information about that person's wishes, values and beliefs. These family members may offer information or be able corroborate what the person themself has reported. They may even be the gatekeepers to enabling an individual to communicate using the required supports or aids, so allowing the person to engage in decision-making.

In other situations, these loved ones may have been identified as *de facto* decision-makers, having been nominated for the role of Lasting Power of Attorney (LPA) or Deputy. This may be a brand new concept for a family member. Indeed, it is not uncommon that health professionals may be involved with the family during the period when they are first applying or being advised to consider this role.

As speech and language therapists (SLTs) working in a social or life participation model, it can be considered our professional responsibility to support people with communication difficulties to access decision-making in all areas of their lives (Ferguson et al., 2010). This chapter will consider the breadth of this role. We will discuss how to explain the MCA (2005) to patients and their families. The role may also involve supporting and advising proxy decision-makers, such as family members, in communication tools and strategies.

Supporting patients and their families during the assessment process

As health professionals, we often assume our patients and their families have more knowledge than they actually do. Equally, we may assume the reverse, that they know less than they actually do. Yet something a health professional considers a well-known fact, such as knowing what some simple parts of the human anatomy look like and how they work, may be a mystery to an otherwise intelligent person. This principle extends to the MCA (2005). Many non-health or non-legal professionals may not even know of its existence, let alone what it says and means.

Thus Graham and Cowley (2015) emphasise that providing guidance on what the MCA (2005) means to a patient and their loved ones is an important part of how "we fully uphold the real opportunities to maximise capacity and support decision-making" (p. 33). Carling-Rowland et al. (2014) elaborate on this by advocating "the right to a fair and just capacity evaluation includes the right to understand that your capacity is being evaluated and the consequences of a finding of incapacity" (p. 761).

Indeed, the MCA Code of Practice (2007) for England and Wales states that:

> "It is important not to assess someone's understanding before they have been given relevant information about a decision." (p. 46)

For some decisions, often the more important, this will include providing information on what the MCA (2005) requires us as health professionals to do. This will include: explaining the need to conduct an assessment of the issue in question; the process by which this occurs; and, for example, that we will be providing information and asking questions about a particular decision in order to assess whether the person is able to understand, retain and weigh up the issues and then communicate their decision. Graham and Cowley (2015) also promote providing information on the need to collect information as part of this assessment, such as details about the person's beliefs and values.

It will also be valuable to ensure that we communicate the outcome of the assessment and the process that will be followed as a consequence, such as a recommendation for the appointment of a Deputy. Graham and Cowley (2015) provide an example of how this can go wrong, describing an individual who has had a stroke who was previously estranged from his wife. They report how the team starts deferring to her for decision-making after his stroke, without involving the preferred advocate named by the patient himself. The authors warn of the confusion and distress that can arise when people are not fully informed of these processes.

Ideally, it is recommended that clinicians spend the time speaking to both the person whom they are assessing, and the loved ones and family around that person. In reality, there is not always the time available in clinical practice to spend time with every relevant loved one or family member to ensure they have fully processed the information given them. It is well understood that people are unlikely to retain every detail from this type of information-giving session fully and completely.

Written leaflets can provide the relevant information for individuals to read and re-visit in their own time. The gov.uk website provides a series of valuable documents including the MCA (2005) process, the MCA Code of Practice (2007) and a series of other related documents. Many people will have found this internet resource themselves, but it is quite complex. There is also a lay summary of the MCA (2005) developed to provide clear information in a plain English format to service users and their carers and family members (Office of the Public Guardian, 2015). This resource attempts to provide information in an accessible format, for example:

> "...your capacity may depend on the type of decision to be made. For example, you may be able to make decisions about day-to-day things, such as what to eat for dinner and what to wear, but be unable to make a decision about financial things, like what to do with your savings." (Office of the Public Guardian, 2015, p. 12)

Additionally, many websites present information related to the (2005) process in a clear, accessible format. Many disease-specific websites present this information for both carers and patients alike (see Table 9.1).

Individual National Health Service (NHS) Trusts may also have leaflets or documents about the MCA (2005). But it may be useful to produce your own aphasia/dementia/brain injury-friendly advice sheets with the support of the MCA lead in your trust. The NIHR has developed a resource to support researchers in engaging people with aphasia (Pearl, 2014). This document advocates using aphasia-friendly research information and consent forms as part of the process of gaining consent from people with aphasia. Yet in clinical practice we rarely produce information leaflets or consent forms, aside from when considering a special situation such as video recording or a video-fluoroscopy X-ray. Chapter 5 provides specific advice on the process of assessing communication to understand the communication requirements for a decision-making assessment. This chapter provides advice on making information accessible. It will be important to consider this when producing an information leaflet on what the MCA (2005) is. This type of innovative yet simple resource is a valuable way to promote and fully maximise the skills of some of our patients and certainly their families; the more they understand, the more likely they will be to demonstrate the skills they have in the assessment process.

Table 9.1 Resource list for accessible advice on what the MCA (2005) is for people and their family members.

NHS Choices website: http://www.nhs.uk/conditions/social-care-and-support-guide/pages/mental-capacity.aspx
Carers UK provides a useful overview of mental capacity: https://www.carersuk.org/help-and-advice/practical-support/managing-someone-s-affairs/mental-capacity
Alzheimer's Society provides a useful overview of mental capacity as well as information on the process of applying for power of attorney: http://www.alzheimers.org.uk/site/scripts/documents_info.php?documentID=354
They also have useful booklet on how to act on behalf of someone with dementia: http://www.alzheimers.org.uk/sharinginformation
Age UK: http://www.ageuk.org.uk/money-matters/legal-issues/powers-of-attorney/mental-capacity/
Age UK has also developed a useful guide on the role of Power of Attorney: http://www.ageuk.org.uk/Documents/EN-GB/Information-guides/AgeUKIG21_Powers_of_attorney_inf.pdf?epslanguage=en-GB?dtrk=true
Headway UK has a fact sheet on the MCA (2005) available on their website, and a booklet about supporting people to make decisions. Both these documents provide information on what the MCA (2005) means and says in a clear accessible way. https://www.headway.org.uk/shop/supporting-people-to-make-decisions.aspx
Mind provide a series of fact sheets on their website about the MCA (2005): http://www.mind.org.uk/information-support/legal-rights/mental-capacity-act-2005/#.VfQm-Ol9nww
Mencap UK also provide a series of useful resources and documents about the MCA (2005): https://www.mencap.org.uk/mental-capacity-act-resource
Other disease-specific organisations may have advice, information or a position on the MCA (2005) available. These may be accessible via the individual relevant third sector organisation website or through directly contacting the organisations.

What can the SLT do to support LPA and Deputies as decision-makers?

Aside from providing information on what the MCA (2005) is, it is important to consider the implications of assessment results. Once we have completed an assessment we should be mindful not to abandon the patient and the family members who may be the potential future decision-makers for that person. Carers and family members of people with communication difficulties can benefit from training to enable them to engage in conversations around daily decision-making (Murphy et al., 2008). When a family member or carer has been established as proxy decision-maker as either an LPA or in a Deputy role, it will be even more important that they understand the process of how to engage their loved ones in these types of conversations.

The MCA Code of Practice (2007) explains that a nominated LPA or Deputy should first consider whether the person could actually make the specific decision him- or herself before embarking on making a decision for them. Considering each issue individually is important, as we know that people do not in general 'globally' lack capacity. Should the person not be able to engage in decision-making, it is still important to ensure they are involved in the decision so they can express their preferences. This will not always be possible in some situations, for example where a carer prevents someone who lacks capacity to understand the danger posed by traffic from stepping out into the middle of a busy road (Office of Public Guardian website, viewed September 2015).

The decisions made on behalf of someone else must be made in their 'best interests'. As explained in Chapter 3, establishing someone's best interests means taking all the relevant factors into account, including the person's previous and current opinions, values, beliefs and choices. "It is perhaps easier to use the word preferences to describe the things people like or dislike, choose or refuse. Some people might only make these preferences known through their behaviour or reactions. Others might point, look or choose from two or three options" (Mencap, 2010/11). Often it is the family and carers who can decipher or understand these behaviours.

Carers UK emphasises that carers probably know more about the person they care for than anyone else, and so want the best for them. Where a carer is also an LPA or Deputy, this can be a great advantage. Yet, they may not always have *all* the strategies and skills to communicate with the person who is recently aphasic, or where their communication is constantly changing and progressing.

What does the law say about how LPAs and Deputys should communicate with their loved ones?

The Scottish Incapacity Act Revised Code of Conduct (2008) includes an Annex focusing on guidance for Attorney decision-makers in communicating with a person with impaired capacity. This Annex includes a series of tips and hints such as:

- Take time to explain to the adult what decision requires to be made and what issues are involved

- Use simple language

- Choose a time of day when the adult is alert and ready for a discussion

- Choose a quiet location where interruptions are unlikely.

(Scottish Government, Revised Code of Practice, 2008, p. 140)

The guidance also advises decision-makers to seek specialist help and advice from an SLT. The MCA Code of Practice (2007) for England and Wales provides similar advice, recommending that LPAs use the guidance set out in Chapter 3 of the MCA Code of Practice (2007) on how to help people make decisions, and seek advice from an SLT where required. Chapter 3 of the MCA Code of Practice (2007) includes guidance similar to the above as well as other more specific statements such as:

- Are mechanical devices such as voice synthesisers, keyboards or other computer equipment available to help?

- If the person does not use verbal communication skills, allow more time to learn how to communicate effectively.

- For people who use nonverbal methods of communication, their behaviour (in particular, changes in behaviour) can provide indications of their feelings.

(England and Wales, MCA Code of Practice, 2007, p. 34)

What does this look like in practice?

Some of the third sector organisations have developed resources for supporting those who are acting in the role of decision-makers such as LPAs. Age UK, Headway and Alzheimer's Society have produced leaflets about how to make decisions on behalf of others (see Table 9.1). The Alzheimer's Society's document entitled "Accessing and sharing information. Acting on behalf of a person with dementia" provides a detailed breakdown of how the process works legally. Booklets published by Age UK and Headway have a similar focus with little guidance on communication. Although it will be helpful to guide people towards these documents they may not cover all their needs. Mencap has developed a resource for relatives of people with learning difficulties on how to keep them involved in decision-making. Although focused on learning disabilities they provide many practical suggestions on communication in their Mental Capacity Resource Pack (Section 8, Mencap website, viewed September 2015) including:

> "You have a lot of information about your relative that will help to keep them at the centre of decision making. This can include communication passports, health action plans and hospital passports. Make sure these are developed and kept up to date. It is hard to ignore somebody that you can see. Think of creative ways to make sure people making decisions know your relative well. This might mean taking them to appointments, showing photos or video clips of them or using any of the communication and health tools described in this pack."

In partnership with the British Institute for Learning Disabilities, Mencap has developed a practical guide, *Involve Me*, to help people with learning disabilities be involved in decision-making. Although this resource is designed for people with learning disabilities, it does provide a useful framework for considering what might be included when training or guiding carers in how to engage anyone with a communication difficulty in decision-making. *Involve Me* includes eight key messages to support people to express their preferences which are easily transferable to people with aphasia, dementia and other communication difficulties.

1. **Know the person really well**: Build on known preferences to support choice, decision-making and consultation. You may know that the person is able to engage in financial decisions to a certain extent; for example, when buying a new television, you may be aware of previous preferences they have had and discuss these with them. People retain many of their pre-stroke or pre-injury preferences, or may form new preferences which carers come to understand. These can be useful when considering a new decision.

2. **Take lots of time**: Take your time, using every opportunity to develop involvement in choice, decision-making and consultation. Don't expect an individual with communication difficulties to be able to engage in a decision within a 5-minute conversation. Supported conversation takes time. It may be that an initial medical appointment where the doctor explained something was just too quick. Yet they will benefit from reading the written information leaflets about a recommended procedure with you at home to be able to engage in discussion on what is going to happen and what it means. Suggesting that people engage in more than one conversation about a decision can help.

3. **Don't make assumptions**: People make assumptions about the communication, levels of involvement and quality of life of others. For example, when considering artificial nutrition or end-of-life decisions, many people assume that their loved one would prefer to stay alive no matter what. It is worth engaging people to ensure they are able to express their preference; it can also be a relief to decision-makers in making difficult decisions. NB: Many serious decisions will need to be taken to the Court of Protection.

4. **Be responsive to the person**: People with communication difficulties are often excluded from decision-making and consultation because it is assumed they have nothing to say. You may be surprised by someone's interest and ability to engage in a decision. Including someone in this process can, in turn, make him or her feel engaged in the decision outcome. It is worth considering reconnecting with an SLT to support you if there is a relatively important decision to be made, such as a large financial decision. SLTs can often support this process and think of new ways to engage the person.

5. **Be creative and try out new ideas**: Working in ways that puts the person with communication difficulties at the centre of the decision-making or consultation process means that they are more likely to feel included. It can also be a challenge to consider how to make the issue clear in a conversation. Writing down key words, drawing pictures, looking at photos of the issue in question can support their understanding and the process of engagement. There may be other means by which they can communicate their preferences, such as gesture and actions, or engaging with high- or low-tech supports that have been designed for the process (e.g. communication books and aids, communication passports, Talking Mats©).

6. **Learn from what the person 'tells' you**: The person with communication difficulties may know and understand more than we realise. Asking the person about what they currently understand about the decision to be made can act as a guide about how you may wish to involve them. There may be instances where people with cognitive difficulties, for example following a brain injury, may attempt to communicate their concerns about issues through irritability, aggression, or other changes in their behaviour. Observe the person to learn what they are telling you.

7. **Act on what you learn**: As we know, people are not labelled as being globally unable to make decisions. Each decision is different. Many decisions may be abstract and difficult to engage with for a person with communication difficulties, especially where finances or complex health matters are concerned. Others may be more tangible and concrete and a person may be able to engage, for example choosing what to wear, where to go today, how to budget small amounts of money in the supermarket. It is important that each time there is a decision to be made we don't assume the person lacks capacity but that we check again.

8. **Help the person recall and share things about their life**: Friends and family members often know the person and their pre-aphasia or pre-dementia experiences. As future carers, they may be better able to remember and recall decision-making experiences that have been made post-brain injury or diagnosis. Sharing stories, particularly about choices, can be a useful tool to engage people and remind them of the process of decision-making. Recording these

in some way can add to these processes in the future. Memory aids or narrative aids such as photos, videos and story telling can enable people in the future.

What does the evidence say about training decision-makers such as LPAs and Deputies?

There is a paucity of research literature in the area of decision-making capacity and communication difficulties, and even less when considering the specific issue of training LPAs and Deputies. There is some emerging literature from specific groups such as the Talking Mats© organisation which is summarised below. There is also a little work being done on training other groups of health professionals such as social workers which can be useful. Indeed, Carling-Rowland et al. (2014) found that social workers made more accurate decisions following specific training on communication, paired with a structured tool to support capacity assessments of people with aphasia. Most convincingly, there is a growing evidence base for the success of training carers and family members as conversation partners for people with aphasia, brain injury and dementia. These types of programmes can form the basis of our training for carers and family members and may be augmented by specific advice around conversations on decision-making.

Using communication aids with carers and their loved ones

Talking Mats© has been described elsewhere in this book as a low-technology communication framework using a simple system of picture symbols that are placed on a textured mat in a particular order to allow people to discuss and indicate their views about various options. Murphy et al. (2010) describe using a scale and inviting individuals with dementia to place images related to a particular topic into this visual scale (see Figure 5.1). For example, if the discussion is around support for daily living, the person can place pictorial images of different activities on a scale, rating them as 'things I can do on my own, things I am unsure about, and things I need support with'.

Murphy and her colleagues have conducted a number of studies into the use of Talking Mats© with people with dementia. In their article published in 2007 they describe a larger-scale research study into the use of Talking Mats© to support communication between unfamiliar listeners and patients with dementia. They used Talking Mats© in conversations to examine how 31 people at different stages of dementia felt about their lives. The researchers determined effectiveness by examining video clips of conversations and rating how much the person with dementia understood, the degree of engagement, their ability to stay on topic, and the degree to which the listener could understand the person with dementia. They found that people could communicate more effectively using Talking Mats© compared to unstructured or semi-structured conversations. They also found that patients produced more reliable information when using Talking Mats© than structured conversation, when information was compared to real-life events. Murphy et al. (2007) made practical recommendations about using Talking Mats© that included the need for personalised images if necessary, and that symbols need to be simple with large text. Finally, they highlighted that some participants may need support in placing pictures.

More recently, Murphy et al. (2010) conducted a similar research study but with 18 couples, again comparing the use of Talking Mats© to 'normal' verbal conversations. People with dementia and their carers were asked to discuss if they were managing or needing support in four aspects of daily living: personal care, getting around, housework and activities. The researchers examined the effectiveness of these conversations using a similar method as previously and found that patients were more engaged in conversations using Talking Mats© than in normal conversations. People with dementia were able to keep on track and perseverate less. They demonstrated more confidence and were often able to take control of the mat. The researcher examining the video was better able to understand the person with dementia when using a Talking Mat©. The researchers also observed an improved conversational balance between couples using Talking Mats© when compared to 'normal conversations'. Murphy et al. (2010) found that carers also felt more listened to in Talking Mats© discussions, and attributed this to the observations that both patients and carers talked more when using Talking Mats©.

Research involving the use of Talking Mats© by people with dementia suggests that the system can help people at different stages of the dementia process and their family carers to feel more involved in discussions that include decision-making, and more satisfied with the outcomes of these discussions (Murphy et al., 2013).

The majority of the literature on communication passports focuses on children in schools and nurseries or adults with learning disabilities, and of these very little research has focused on decision-making capacity issues. This literature is only emerging and frequently focuses on consent for research. An example of this is a study by Calveley (2012) who describes the methods that were used to enable people with severe and profound intellectual disabilities, who lacked capacity, to participate in a study that examined their experience of receiving intimate care. They introduced communication passports as a method for engaging people in the consent process. The researchers describe how communication passports contained easily accessible information that enabled people to understand and interpret nonverbal communication. Communication passports are often used and recommended for adults, particularly those with progressive conditions such as dementia, multiple sclerosis or motor neurone disease.

In Northern Ireland (NI), the Royal College of General Practitioners NI was commissioned by the Public Health Agency NI to create a tool for patients with progressive, life-limiting illness such as dementia or any other progressive neurological condition, their families and carers. The aim of the tool was to improve the collection, availability and reliability of clinical information associated with patients. This research work focused on consulting with patients, patient advocate groups, carers, and professional colleagues about the form that the 'End-of-Life Care Passport' might take. They found that individuals and carers rejected the concept of an 'End-of-Life Care Passport', as being focused on difficulties and limitations rather than on abilities and wellbeing. The groups identified that the life journey with progressive illness may require a communication passport throughout, which would be updated and adapted as an on-going process. They also found the needs of the person and their carers were very different to those of healthcare professionals. They recommend that a communication passport needs to have the person and their carer as the focus for its development (Abbott, 2014; Abbott et al., 2015).

Bourgeois (2007) has published a manual describing the types and formats of different communication aids that can be used with people with dementia. Bourgeois et al. (2009) also briefly describe this manual and summarise a number of studies the authors themselves have carried out examining the use of communication books in conversation between patients with dementia and their caregivers. They report reduced repetitiveness, increased information exchange and reduced ambiguity in conversations when using communication books. They also report increased balance in turn taking and topic maintenance as well as reduced need for partner prompting. Perhaps one of the most useful for residential settings was the finding of enhanced cooperation and reduced problem behaviours when communication aids or memory books were used with care routines. In summarising these studies, they also highlight some of the limitations, particularly the cost and time required to train so many staff members in these specific approaches.

Conversation and communication training

To my knowledge, there is no research evidence on communication training for people in the role of LPA or Deputy. There is, however, some emerging research that highlights the added value of communication training for people who are considered expert assessors of mental capacity. In developing an assessment tool for assessing capacity, Carling-Rowland et al. (2014) also developed a training DVD for the social workers they were working with. The training DVD focused on the effective administration of the tool (the CACE, described more fully in Chapter 4) and communication techniques that were used. An individual with Broca's aphasia of moderate-to-severe severity and a SLT trained in Supported Conversation for Adults with Aphasia (SCATM) (Kagan et al., 2001) participated in the training DVD. The two participants were filmed administering the tool, followed by a conversation that illustrated different supported conversation techniques. The researchers found social workers' performance and accuracy in judging capacity improved with this training.

It is well recognised that SLTs are optimally placed to provide advice and training to carers and family members on communicating with their loved ones with aphasia (Lock et al, 2008; Beeke et al., 2013; Simmons-Mackie et al., 2014). Similarly, the literature is emerging on conversation training for people with brain injuries and their conversation partners (Togher et al., 2013), progressive conditions such as Parkinson's disease (Forsgren et al., 2013), and dementia and their conversation partners (Volkmer, 2013; Volkmer, 2015).

Simmons-Mackie et al. (2014) provide a thorough overview of conversation training for people with aphasia in their review of the literature in this area. Many SLTs will be very familiar with programmes such as Supporting Partners of People with Aphasia in Relationships and Conversation (SPPARC; Lock et al., 2008) and Better Conversation with Aphasia (BCA; Beeke et al., 2013). These programmes have in common individualised feedback on facilitators and barriers to communication (often video-based), followed by strategy training, with the aim of maximising the success of everyday conversations (Simmons-Mackie et al., 2014). Both the SPPARC and BCA guide the SLT on how patients and communication partners can participate in creating and evaluating a video of themselves in conversation, identifying areas of strength and difficulty (such as strategies that worked well or failed), and then problem solving how to improve this interaction, setting goals around this, before trialling strategies together. BCA is a free online package consisting of a therapy manual, video samples and training materials for SLTs and is available at https://extend.ucl. ac.uk/. BCA (Beeke et al., 2013) has a growing evidence base for its ability to significantly change the conversation skills of people with post-stroke aphasia as well as their conversation partners (Beeke et al., 2015; Beeke et al., 2014; Best et al., forthcoming). Video feedback about communication strengths and barriers is believed to be a key facilitator of improved conversational skill. It has been identified that, whilst conversation partner awareness is important, a key mechanism to promote change is actually understanding the *impact* of communication behaviours on the person with aphasia (Johnson, 2015).

Another method of assessment and feedback is the Conversation Analysis Profile for People with Cognitive Impairment (CAPPCI) developed by Perkins et al. (1997) for people with aphasia. It has also been used to good effect with people with dementia and their family members (Perkins et al., 1998). This model of assessment and intervention requires first of all an interview with the caregiver as well as an analysis of a sample of conversation. This information is analysed and combined to provide a profile of what is occurring in interaction. This then supports the planning of appropriate therapy tasks to improve interaction. The interview with the caregiver asks them to rate the frequency of different behaviours. It also allows the clinician to gather information about the type of strategies the caregiver feels they use, as well as how successful these are in practice. The interview attempts to identify whether the carer feels each of the identified behaviours is causing a problem. Finally, the interview also asks about pre-injury versus current communication styles and opportunities for communication. This can guide the amount of education the carer may benefit from. It will also illustrate whether carers have accepted behaviours and whether they may be underestimating their partner's skills. Therapists can reinforce successful strategy use or discourage unsuccessful strategies by comparing the carer report to the conversation sample, as well as highlight unnoticed strategies and suggest new ones.

It has long been recognised that training caregivers of people with brain injuries could be useful. Indeed, in 1993 Ylvisaker described the importance of role playing and modelling combined with ongoing coaching and support in vivo as useful for carers of people with TBI. Since then, researchers such as Togher et al. (2004) have developed and trialled techniques for communication training. Togher et al. (2009) developed a programme called TBI Express for people with TBI and their partners, described further in McDonald et al. (2013), which they compared to providing therapy for the person with TBI alone. TBI Express focuses on teaching conversation partners how to facilitate conversation with the person with a TBI over 10 weeks by, for example, using positive, non-demanding questions, encouraging discussion of opinions and working through difficult communication. They identify the ingredients for successful conversation as collaborative intent (we are in this together), cognitive and emotional support (I am with you, it's OK), positive question style (I am interested) and collaborative turn taking (sharing). TBI Express has been published and has a free website including some demonstration videos at http://sydney.edu.au/health-sciences/tbi-express/. Togher et al. (2014) concluded that the TBI Express condition demonstrated better outcomes for communication, social skills, carer burden and self-esteem than when carers were not included.

The literature in dementia is in some ways quite well developed when considering generic psychosocial supports and some of the more didactic nursing and caregiver communication training. What is only now emerging is the individualised communication training approach that is so valuable in ensuring enduring and more significant outcomes. The RCSLT dementia position paper (2014) advocates that, by providing support and recommending communication strategies, SLTs facilitate the maintenance of relationships. The NICE/SCIE guidelines for dementia (2011) describe how "communication strategies adapted to the individual's needs and abilities are the main building blocks to maximising skills and ensuring the least amount of dependency in care". A recent systematic review of communication skills training for healthcare professionals and family caregivers of people with dementia concluded that such training significantly improves the quality of life and wellbeing of people with dementia and increases positive interactions in various care settings (Eggenberger et al., 2013). In addition, training carers of people with dementia in psychosocial coping strategies is effective in improving their mood and ratings of quality of life (see, for example, the START programme, Livingstone et al., 2013). Despite their efficacy, the majority of these interventions do not actively involve the person with dementia, whose cognition is a barrier to participation. Yet SLTs do report using conversation training for people with PPA and their families (Volkmer, 2015) and there are some single-case studies in the literature where researchers used tools such as the CAPPCI, described above, to guide conversation training with a person with PPA (Wong et al.,

2009) or an adaptation of BCA (Beeke et al., 2013) developed specifically for people with primary progressive aphasia (see Volkmer & Beeke, 2015).

Conclusion

SLTs, families and carers are all responsible for ensuring the MCA (2005) is implemented. Excellent care can only be achieved by remaining constantly mindful of people's best interests and endeavouring to achieve a greater understanding around the person's needs. Ignorance of the law is no defence and a failure to comply with the MCA (2005) may well establish a breach of duty or care owed by a carer. Yet families and carers may benefit from our support in developing their skills in this area to use with people with communication difficulties.

As SLTs, we are well placed to provide communication training for people with communication difficulties and their communication partners or *de facto* decision-makers. This training should, where relevant, provide additional advice on the relevance of communication to decision-making. The MCA (2005) really does put the person at the centre of decisions, just as SLTs ordinarily put people at the centre of a conversation, thus this training is nothing new. It is a skill we have long been honing in the SLT profession.

References

Abbott, A. (2014) Communication and Continuity in Progressive, Life-Limiting Illness. A Report by the Royal College of General Practitioners Northern Ireland: http://www.rcgp.org.uk/rcgp-near-you/rcgp-northern-ireland/~/media/Files/RCGP-Faculties/Northern-Ireland/RCGP-Healthcare-Communication-report.ashx

Abbott, A., Watson, M., Gingles, J., Brown, S., Brennan, J., Scott, K. & Healy, M. (2015) PA10 What i need you to know. Building a collaborative communication tool. *BMJ Supportive & Palliative Care*, 5, A22–A22.

Beeke, S. (2015) Conversation partner training: What is it and does it work? Key Note Presentation: British Aphasiology Society Conference, UCL.

Beeke, S., Sirman, N., Beckley, F., Maxim, J., Edwards, S., Swinburn, K. & Best, W. (2013) Better Conversations with Aphasia: An e-learning resource. Available at: https://extend.ucl.ac.uk/

Beeke, S., Johnson, F., Beckley, F., Heilemann, C., Edwards, S., Maxim, J. & Best, W. (2014) Enabling better conversations between a man with aphasia and his conversation partner: Incorporating writing into turn taking. *Research on Language and Social Interaction*, 47(3): 292–305. DOI: 10.1080/08351813.2014.925667

Beeke, S., Beckley, F., Johnson, F., Heilemann, C., Edwards, S., Maxim, J. & Best, W. (2015) Conversation focused aphasia therapy: Investigating the adoption of strategies by people with agrammatism. *Aphasiology*, 29(3): 355–377 DOI:10.1080/02687038.2014.881459.

Best, W., Beckley, F., Edwards, S., Heilemann, C., Howard, D., Johnson, F., Maxim, J. & Beeke, S. (forthcoming) Investigating the effect of therapy with people with aphasia and conversation partners: A mixed methods group and case series study. *Journal of Speech Language Hearing Research*.

Bourgeois, M.S. (2007) *Memory Books and Other Graphic Cuing Systems*. New York: Health Professions Press, Brookes.

Bourgeois, M.S. & Hickey, E.M. (2009) *Dementia: From Diagnosis to Management - A Functional Approach*. New York: Psychology Press.

Calveley, J. (2012). Including adults with intellectual disabilities who lack capacity to consent in research. *Nursing Ethics*, 19(4): 558–567.

Carers UK website (viewed September 2015):

https://www.carersuk.org/help-and-advice/practical-support/managing-someone-s-affairs/mental-capacity

Carling-Rowland, A., Black, S., McDonald, L. & Kagan, A. (2014) Increasing access to fair capacity evaluation for discharge decision-making for people with aphasia: A randomized controlled trial. *Aphasiology*, 28(6): 750–765.

Eggenberger, E., Heimerl, K. & Bennett, M.I. (2013) Communication skills training in dementia care: A systematic review of effectiveness, training content, and didactic methods in different care settings. *International Psychogeriatrics*, 25(3): 345–358.

Forsgren, E., Antonsson, M. & Saldert, C. (2013) Training conversation partners of persons with communication disorders related to Parkinson's disease—a protocol and a pilot study. *Logopedics Phoniatrics Vocology*, 38(2): 82–90.

Ferguson, A., Duffield, G. & Worrall, L. (2010) Legal decision-making by people with aphasia: Critical incidents for speech pathologists. *International Journal of Language & Communication Disorders*, 45(2): 244–258.

Graham, M. & Cowley, J. (2015) *A Practical Guide to the Mental Capacity Act 2005: Putting the principles of the Act into practice*. London, Jessica Kingsley.

Coping with communication problems after brain injury (Headway, 2014). Available at: https://www.headway.org.uk/shop.aspx

Johnson, F. (2015) What works in conversation therapy for aphasia and how? Searching for mechanisms of change and active ingredients using tools and theory from behaviour change research. Unpublished PhD Thesis, University College London.

Kagan, A., Black, S.E., Duchan, J.F., Simmons-Mackie, N. & Square, P. (2001) Training volunteers as conversation partners using supported conversation for adults with aphasia (SCA) A controlled trial. *Journal of Speech, Language, and Hearing Research*, 44(3): 624–638.

Livingston, G., Barber, J., Rapaport, P., Knapp, M., Griffin, M., King, D., Livingston, D., Mummery, C., Walker, Z., Hoe, J., Sampson, E.L. & Cooper, C. (2013) Clinical effectiveness of a manual based coping strategy programme (START, STrAtegies for RelaTives) in promoting the mental health of carers of family members with dementia: pragmatic randomised controlled trial. *BMJ* , 347: f6276.

McDonald, S., Togher, L. & Code, C. (2013). *Social and Communication Disorders Following Traumatic Brain Injury*. Brighton, Psychology Press.

Mencap (viewed on website September 2015) Mental Capacity Act resource pack. For family carers of people with a learning disability https://www.mencap.org.uk/sites/default/files/documents/mental%20capacity%20act%20resource%20pack.pdf

Mencap, BILD and The Renton Foundation (2010/2011) InvolveMe. Increasing the involvement of people with profound and multiple learning disabilities (PMLD) in decision-making and consultation. https://www.mencap.org.uk/sites/default/files/documents/Involve%20me%20Summary%20Booklet.pdf

Murphy J. & Oliver, T.M. (2013) The use of Talking Mats to support people with dementia and their carers to make decisions together. *Health & Social Care in the Community*, 21((2): 171–180.

Murphy, J., Gray, C.M. & Cox, S. (2007) Talking Mats: The effectiveness of a low technology communication framework to help people with dementia express their views. *Journal of Assistive Technologies*, 1(2): 30–34.

Murphy, J., Oliver, T.M. & Cox S. (2010) Talking Mats and Involvement in Decision Making for People with Dementia and Family Carers: Full Report. Joseph Rowntree Foundation. www.jrf.org.uk. Downloaded from: http://www.jrf,org.uk/sites/files/jrf/Talking-Mats-and-decision-making-full.pdf

National Collaborating Centre for Mental Health commissioned by the Social Care Institute for Excellence National Institute for Health and Clinical Excellence (revised 2011) THE NICE -SCIE GUIDELINE ON SUPPORTING PEOPLE WITH DEMENTIA AND THEIR CARERS IN HEALTH AND SOCIAL CARE, National Clinical Practice Guideline Number 42 published by The British Psychological Society and Gaskell. Downloaded from: http:// www.nice.org.uk/nicemedia/live/10998/30320/30320.pdf

Office of Public Guardian (website viewed September 2015) Making decisions about your health, welfare or finances. Who decides when you can't? Department of Health UK: https://www.gov.uk/government/uploads/system/uploads/attachment_data/file/365631/making_decisions-opg601.pdf

Pearl, G. (2014) Engaging with people who have aphasia: A set of resources for stroke researchers. NIHR CRN: Stroke

Perkins, L., Whitworth, A. & Lesser, R. (1998). Conversing in dementia: A conversation analytic approach. *Journal of Neurolinguistics*, 11(1), 33–53.

Royal College of Speech and Language Therapists (2014) Speech and Language Therapy Provision for people with dementia. RCSLT Position Paper. http://www.rcslt.org/members/publications/publications2/dementia_position_paper2014

Scottish Government (2008) Revised Code of Practice for persons authorised under intervention orders and guardians. Scotland. RR Donnelley. http://www.gov.scot/Resource/Doc/216558/0058064.pdf

Social Care Institute for Excellence guidance on accessible information: http://www.scie.org.uk/publications/misc/accessguidelinespublications.asp

Simmons-Mackie, N. Savage, M.C. & Worrall, L. (2014) Conversation therapy for aphasia: A qualitative review of the literature. *Internantional Journal of Language and Communication Disorders*, 49(5): 511–526.

Talking Mats information and resources: http://www.talkingmats.com/

Togher, L., McDonald, S., Code, C. & Grant, S. (2004) Training communication partners of people with traumatic brain injury: A randomised controlled trial. *Aphasiology*, 18(4): 313–335.

Togher, L., McDonald, S., Tate, R., Power, E. & Rietdijk, R. (2009) Training communication partners of people with traumatic brain injury: Reporting the protocol for a clinical trial. *Brain Impairment*, 10(02): 188–204.

Togher, L., McDonald, S., Tate, R., Power, E. & Riedtijk, R. (2013) Training communication partners of people with severe traumatic brain injury improves everyday conversations: A multicenter single blind clinical trial. *Journal of Rehabilitation Medicine*, 45, 637–645.

Togher, L., McDonald, S., Tate, R., Power, E. & Rietdijk, R. (2014) Training everyday communication partners is efficacious in improving the communication of people with severe TBI: Findings from a single-blind multi-center clinical trial. *Brain Injury*, 28(5–6): 723–724.

Volkmer, A. (2013) *Assessment and Therapy for Language and Cognitive Communication Difficulties in Dementia and Other Progressive Diseases*. Guildford, J&R Press.

Volkmer, A. (2015) Communication training keeps families together. *Bulletin*, 756.

Volkmer, A. & Beeke, S. (2015) How to help couples have better conversations. *Journal of Dementia Care*, 23(5): 22–24.

Wong, S.B., Anand, R., Chapman, S.B., Rackley, A. & Zientz, J. (2009) When nouns and verbs degrade: Facilitating communication in semantic dementia. *Aphasiology*, 23(2): 286–301.

Ylvisaker, M. (1993) Communication outcome in children and adolescents with traumatic brain injury. *Neuropsychological Rehabilitation*, 3(4): 367–387.

Afterword

Public interest in decision-making capacity is increasing. Since the Mental Capacity Act (2005) was introduced, speech and language therapists (SLTs) have become increasingly more involved with the process of assessing decision-making. This involvement remains variable depending on the setting, the service and the team. It is now, however, indisputable that SLTs need to be involved in this process so that people with communication difficulties are able to have a voice in decision-making in relation to their own lives. This is their right.

The processes surrounding decision-making, such as advance care planning outlined in the MCA (2005), can also significantly influence management decisions for a person with dysphagia or a person with communication difficulties. We need to keep informed about this legislation and how this can impact upon the care we provide.

Resources

The information in this book will quickly become out of date. Use your team and the local services such as the MCA representative in your Trust to keep you updated. The following websites may also be useful resources to consult for updates and advice.

Useful contacts for patients

Age UK: http://www.ageuk.org.uk/money-matters/legal-issues/powers-of-attorney/mental-capacity/

Age UK has also developed a useful guide about the role of Power of Attorney:

http://www.ageuk.org.uk/Documents/EN-GB/Information-guides/AgeUKIG21_Powers_of_attorney_inf.pdf?epslanguage=en-GB?dtrk=true

Alzheimer's Society website information sheet: http://www.alzheimers.org.uk/site/scripts/documents_info.php?documentID=354

They also produce a useful booklet on how to act of behalf of someone with dementia: http://www.alzheimers.org.uk/sharinginformation

Carers UK provides a useful overview of mental capacity: https://www.carersuk.org/help-and-advice/practical-support/managing-someone-s-affairs/mental-capacity

Compassion in Dying website and advance care planning resources:

http://compassionindying.org.uk/making-decisions-and-planning-your-care/planning-ahead/advance-decisions-to-refuse-treatment/

Headway UK has a fact sheet about the MCA (2005) available on its website, and you can also buy a booklet on supporting people to make decisions. Both these documents provide information on what the MCA (2005) means and says in a clear, accessible way. https://www.headway.org.uk/shop/supporting-people-to-make-decisions.aspx

Mencap UK provides a series of useful resources and documents about the MCA (2005): https://www.mencap.org.uk/mental-capacity-act-resource

Mind website summary: http://www.mind.org.uk/information-support/legal-rights/mental-capacity-act-2005/#.VcN8Tet9nwx

NHS website: http://www.nhs.uk/Conditions/social-care-and-support-guide/Pages/mental-capacity.aspx

Useful resource contacts for clinicians

Mental Capacity Act 2005: http://www.legislation.gov.uk/ukpga/2005/9/contents

Mental Capacity assessment audit tool: http://www.amcat.org.uk

Social Care Institute of Excellence website information: http://www.scie.org.uk/publications/mca/index.asp

Social Care Institute of Excellence online training resources: http://www.scie.org.uk/mca-directory/trainingcourses.asp

An excellent website which provides links to other websites and updates on case law is: http://www.mentalcapacitylawandpolicy.org.uk/resources-2/

Index